Veterinary Andrology & Artificial Insemination

(For the Students of B.V.Sc. & A.H. Degree Programme)

Veterinary Andrology & Artificial Insemination

(For the Students of B.V.Sc. & A.H. Degree Programme)

M.S.Saxena

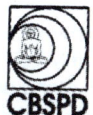

CBS Publishers & Distributors Pvt Ltd

New Delhi • Bengaluru • Chennai • Kochi • Kolkata • Lucknow • Mumbai
Hyderabad • Jharkhand • Nagpur • Patna • Pune • Uttarakhand

Veterinary Andrology and Artificial Insemination

ISBN: 978-81-239-0716-1

First Edition: 2000
Reprint: 2004, 2007, 2011, 2012, 2013, 2015, 2020, 2021, 2023, 2024

Published by **Satish Kumar Jain** and produced by **Varun Jain** for

CBS Publishers & Distributors Pvt Ltd
4819/XI Prahlad Street, 24 Ansari Road, Daryaganj, New Delhi 110 002, India.
Ph: 011-23289259, 23266861

Website: www.cbspd.com
e-mail: delhi@cbspd.com

Corporate Office: 204 FIE, Industrial Area, Patparganj, Delhi 110 092
Ph: 011-4934 4934

Fax: 011-4934 4935 e-mail: publishing@cbspd.com; publicity@cbspd.com

Branches

- **Bengaluru:** Seema House 2975, 17th Cross, K.R. Road, Banasankari 2nd Stage, Bengaluru 560 070, Karnataka, India
  Ph: +91-80-26771678/79   Fax: +91-80-26771680   e-mail: bangalore@cbspd.com
- **Chennai:** 7, Subbaraya Street, Shenoy Nagar, Chennai 600 030, Tamil Nadu, India
  Ph: +91-44-26680620, 26681266   Fax: +91-44-42032115   e-mail: chennai@cbspd.com
- **Kochi:** 42/1325, 1326, Power House Road, Opp KSEB, Ernakulam 682 018, Kochi, Kerala, India
  Ph: +91-484-4059061-67   Fax: +91-484-4059065   e-mail: kochi@cbspd.com
- **Kolkata:** 147, Hind Ceramics Compound, 1st Floor, Nilgunj Road, Belghoria, Kolkata 700 056, West Bengal, India
  Ph: +91-33-25633055/56   e-mail: kolkata@cbspd.com
- **Lucknow:** Basement, Khushnuma Complex, 7-Meerabai Marg (Behind Jawahar Bhawan), Lucknow 226 001, UP, India
  Ph: +0552-4000032   e-mail: tiwari.lucknowi@cbspd.com
- **Mumbai:** PWD Shed. Gala no. 25/26, Ramchandra Bhatt Marg, Next to JJ Hospital Gate no. 2, Opp. Union Bank of India, Noorbaug, Mumbai 400 009, Maharashtra, India
  Ph: 022-66661880/89   e-mail: mumbai@cbspd.com

Representatives

• **Hyderabad**	0-9885175004	• **Jharkhand**	0-9811541605	• **Nagpur**	0-8692091830
• **Patna**	0-9334159340	• **Pune**	0-9664372571	• **Uttarakhand**	0-9716462459

Printed at: Glorious Printers, Delhi, India

Foreword

There is a great paucity of textbooks in the field of veterinary sciences written by Indian authors as reference and textbooks suitable to Indian college curriculum. Most Indian teachers use textbooks written by American and European authors directed at the clientele in their respective countries which are supplemented by notes to suit experience of Indian and other developing countries. This is a very unsatisfactory situation. In spite of a number of efforts by Indian Council of Agricultural Research and the publishing community at large, the number of authors who have taken up the challenge of writing books to serve as textbooks in veterinary colleges are very few. There seems to be no tradition which could generate a crop of authors who could take upon themselves the very important task of writing textbooks suitable for our curriculum in the veterinary colleges.

With the notification of standards for veterinary education by the Indian Veterinary Council, the entire course curriculum has been revised/updated and it is therefore necessary that attempts should be made by various university teachers to prepare texts to suit this course curriculum. Dr. Saxena's attempt to produce a basic text on andrology and artificial insemination based on the syllabus prescribed by Indian Veterinary Council is a good attempt in this direction. The need for a comprehensive book on clinical andrology and artificial insemination meant for undergraduates in the veterinary schools was urgent; this book can now be used as a textbook which will fill the long felt need in the subject. The text is primarily devoted to andrological examination of breeding bulls and their management, collection, evaluation and preservation of semen particularly of buffaloes. This is going to be very useful to the beginners. A chapter on cleaning and sterilization of equipment, recording of data is important from the point of view of veterinary practice. I believe that this compendium will be used as a workbook by the teachers as well as students. They should assist Dr. Saxena in improving its functional use in due course of time.

P.N. Bhat
Chairman, World Buffalo Trust

v

Preface

Reproduction is a joint venture in which both males and females participate. Reproductive disorders are more apparent in females, hence failures are often attributed to female gender only. A close examination of the process, however, reveals that males are as great offenders as females to cause infertility problems. The male should provide sperms which are competent to fertilize the ovum. Whenever there is large-scale problem of infertility in a herd or in large number of females, the male is always seen with suspicion. In addition to productive efficiency, the clinical examination of the bull for its reproductive efficiency is gaining more and more popularity.

There are many excellent books on andrology and A.I. which would undoubtedly remain unmatched for many years to come. None of these are tailor-made for the B.V.Sc. & A.H. syllabus prescribed by Indian Veterinary Council and followed by Indian veterinary institutions. Necessity for a concise book on "Clinical Andrology and A.I." within the scope and apprehension of undergraduate veterinary students has thus been felt for long. This compendium cum workbook has been attempted with the expectation that it would fulfill this long felt need and would provide necessary guidelines to the B.V.Sc. & A.H. students.

Basically, the contents of the book have been drawn from diverse literary sources as well as the practical field experience of the author. There might be some errors in the text and there is tremendous scope for improvement. The suggestions and criticisms would always be heartily welcomed.

Many of my senior colleagues, my associates, friends and students have made valuable contributions towards compilation of this book and the author is deeply indebted to Dr. Harpal Singh, Dean, College of Veterinary Sciences; Dr. S.N. Maurya, Prof. & Head, Department of Gynaecology and Obstetrics; Dr. B.D. Lakhchaura, Prof. & Head, Department of Veterinary Biochemistry for their inspiration and valuable suggestions. Dr. V. Umapathi, Junior Research Officer and Mr. K.C. Joshi, Steno-typist of the Department of Veterinary Biochemistry deserve exceptional appreciation for their wholehearted help. Sincere thanks are due to Dr. V.B. Saxena, Dr. H.P. Gupta and Dr. Shiv Prasad for their critical suggestions. Km. Geeta Kandpal, Teaching Associate of the Department of Veterinary Biochemistry deserves appreciation in handling work on computer. The author would like to express his appreciation and indebtedness to his wife Meena and daughters, Shilpi and Shubhangi for their understanding and forgiveness they had shown for his several long absences from home.

M.S. Saxena

Syllabus (For B.V.Sc. & A.H. Degree Programme)

Andrology and Artificial Insemination

VOG-511   **Cr. Hrs. 2 + 0 = 2**

Introduction, development, comparative study of male genitalia and gonads. Growth, puberty, sexual maturity and libido. Endocrine control of reproduction in the male domestic animals. Factors affecting maturity and sex drive in bulls. Sexual behaviour in males. Forms of male infertility. General considerations. Factors affecting infertility in male, its treatment and diagnosis. Diseases, abnormalities and malformations of male genitalia, their diagnosis and treatment of coital injury and infections. Testicular hypoplasia and degeneration. Diseases of the accessory sex glands. Introduction, history, development, advantages and limitations of A.I. methods of semen collection in various species. Technique of A.I. factors affecting quality and quantity of semen. Tests for evaluation of semen; extension of semen; preservation of semen at different temperatures. Storage and shipment of semen, metabolism of semen, biochemistry of semen.

Andrology and Artificial Insemination (Clinics)

VOG-512   **Cr. Hrs. 0 + 2 :: 2**

Andrological investigations of breeding bulls. Assessment of sires. Physical examinations—observing sexual behaviour; palpation of scrotum, spermatic cord, seminal vesicles and ampullae. Collection of materials for sperm activity, morphology and diagnosis of reproductive disorders in bulls. Preparation of A.V., collection of semen, evaluation, dilution, preservation techniques at different temperature. Freezing of semen. Insemination techniques in chilled and frozen semen. Planning and organization of A.I. centre. Selection, care, training and maintenance of breeding bulls for A.I., recording systems. Care, sterilization. Storage and upkeep of equipments used for Artificial Insemination.

Contents

SECTION I

SECTION II

EXERCISES

Chapter 1

Reproductive Organs of Male Domestic Animals

The male reproductive organs consist of two testes (or testicles) which are contained in the scrotum, ducts, accessory sex glands and the penis. The reproductive organs of the bulls are shown in Fig. 1.1 and the comparative anatomy of the male reproductive organs of different domestic animals is illustrated in Fig. 1.2.

The testis produces spermatozoa and the male sex hormone (testosterone). The scrotum helps in maintaining optimum temperature for the spermatozoa production. The other structures help for the passage of .he spermatozoa to the site of deposition in the female's genitalia in a fairly good condition that may lead to fertilization of the ovum/ova.

SCROTUM AND TESTES

The scrotum is a cutaneous pouch (derived from the skin and fascia) in which testicles are located. The scrotum in all the domestic animals except in boar and cat is located in between thighs. In boar and cat the scrotum is located caudal to thighs. The testis is fixed to the scrotum by means of scrotal ligament attached to its caudal end near the tail of the epididymis. The hairs on the scrotum are very scantly present. Different layer of tissues that are present in between the scrotal skin and the testis proper are shown in Fig. 1.3.

1. **Tunica dartos layer** is present under the scrotal skin and is composed of smooth muscle fibers with fibrous and elastic connective tissue. Tunica dartos layer surrounds both the testes and forms a medial septum in between two testes.

2. **Loose connective tissue layer** is present under the tunica dartos layer.

3. **Vaginal process layer** is present under the loose connective tissue layer. Vaginal process is an extension of peritoneum passing through the abdominal wall at the inguinal canal. The vaginal process layer is composed of (a) superficial layer called tunica vaginalis communis, which corresponds to the parietal peritoneum of the abdominal cavity; and (b) deeper layer called tunica vaginalis propria, which corresponds the visceral layer of peritoneum of the abdominal cavity.

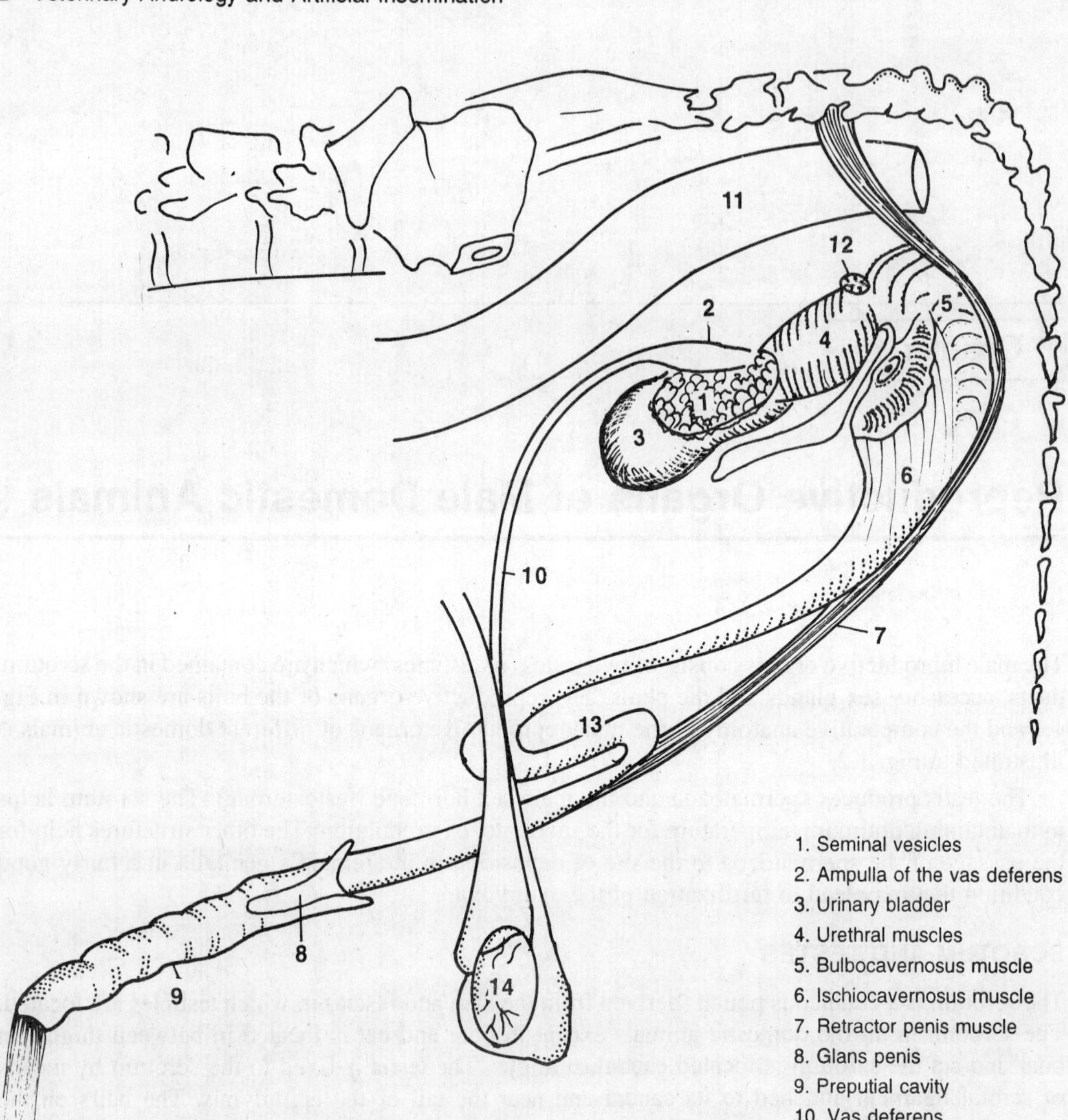

1. Seminal vesicles
2. Ampulla of the vas deferens
3. Urinary bladder
4. Urethral muscles
5. Bulbocavernosus muscle
6. Ischiocavernosus muscle
7. Retractor penis muscle
8. Glans penis
9. Preputial cavity
10. Vas deferens
11. Rectum
12. Bulbourethral gland
13. Sigmoid flexure
14. Testis

Fig. 1.1. Reproductive organs of the bull.

4. **Tunica albuginea layer** is the tough layer composed of fibromuscular tissue present beneath the visceral layer of the vaginal process.

Extensions of the tunica albuginea penetrate the testicular parenchyma to join at mediastinum. Fibrous septa divided the testicular parenchyma into lobules containing the highly coiled seminiferous tubules. About 75% of the testicular mass is composed of seminiferous tubules. The length of the seminiferous tubules estimated in different species is as follows :

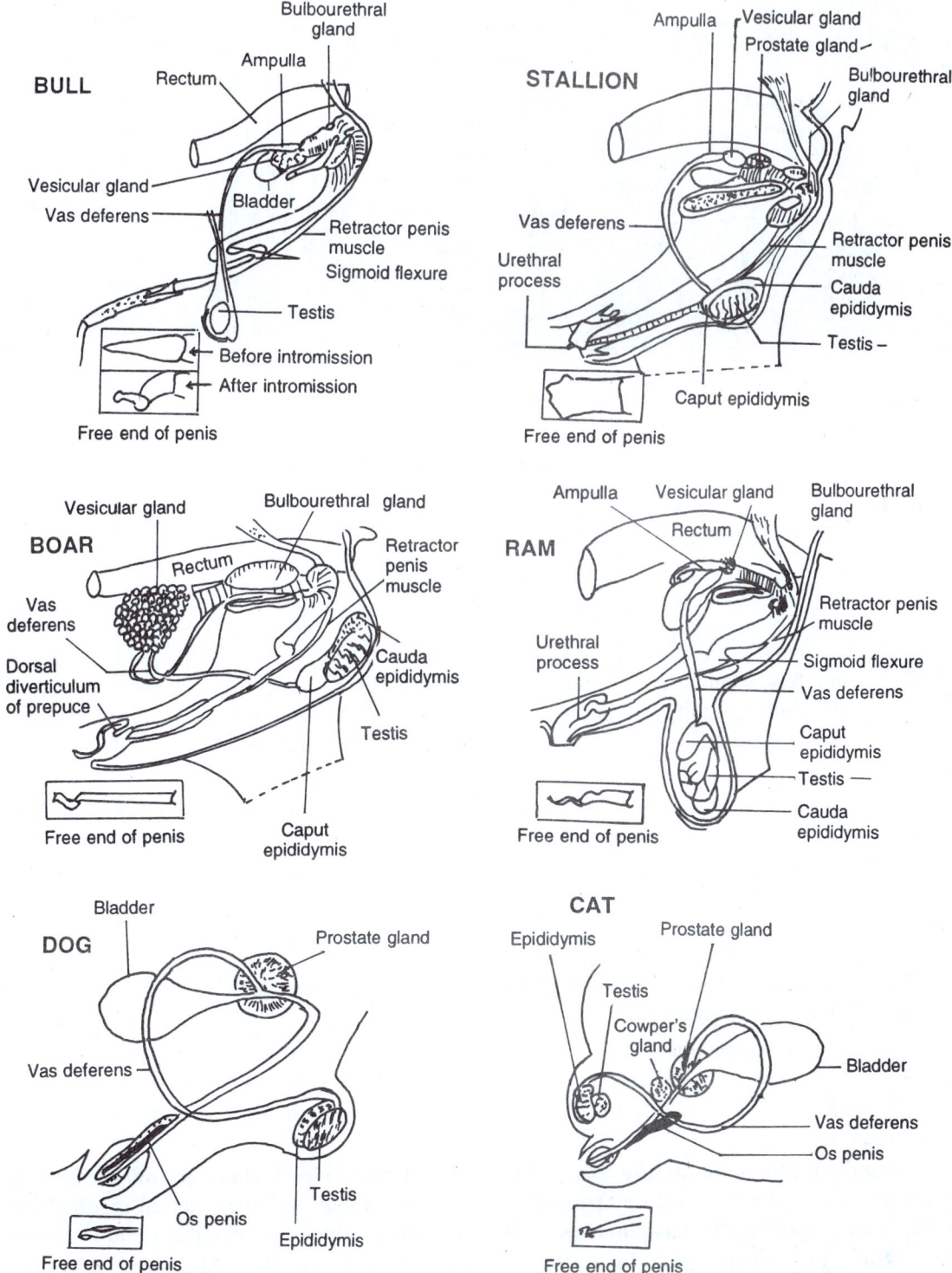

Fig. 1.2. Diagrams showing comparative anatomy of male reproductive organs of bull, stallion, boar, ram, dog and cat.

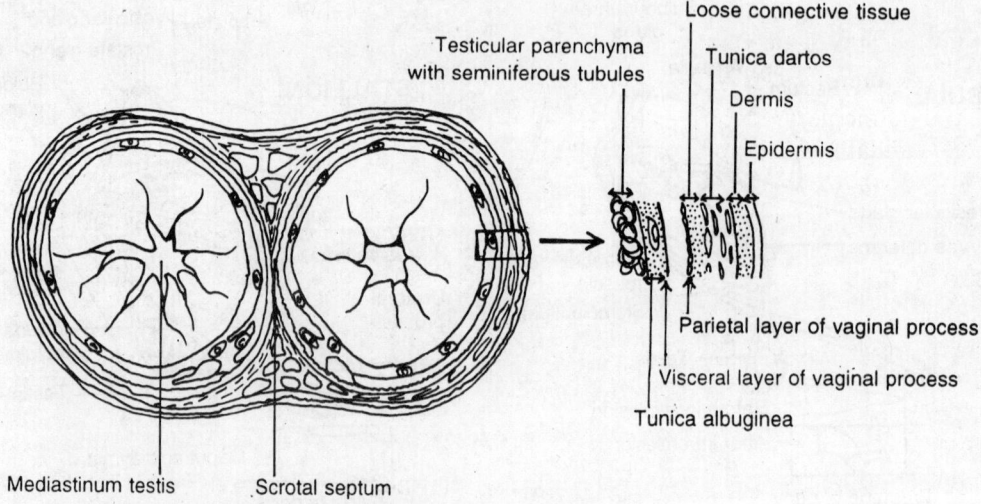

Fig. 1.3. Schematic horizontal section through scrotum to show different layers.

Bull	5000 m
Ram	4000 m
Boar	6000 m
Dog	150 m
Cat	25 m

The seminiferous tubules are lined by germinal epithelium and produce spermatozoa. The seminiferous tubules join the rete testes through straight tubules (the tubuli recti). From rete testes the sperm cells are passed to efferent tubules (6 to 24 in number) and than to head of the epididymis (Fig. 1.4).

In stallion there is no mediastinum testes and the collecting tubules join the efferent tubules. Thus in bull the passage of the spermatozoa from seminiferous tubules is as follows :

Seminiferous tubules → Tubuli recti → Rete testes → Efferent tubules

↓

Urethra ← Ampulla ← Vas deferens ← Epididymis

The testis in the scrotal pouch is held by its tunics and the spermatic cord. The spermatic cord is composed of the following :

1. Internal spermatic artery.

Vaginal process is an extension of the peritoneum passing through abdominal wall at the inguinal canal.

Inguinal canal is the slit like space between the internal abdominal oblique muscle forming the internal inguinal ring (deep opening of the inguinal canal) and the external inguinal ring (superficial opening of the inguinal canal) formed by the tendon of the external oblique muscle.

Rut is the certain definite period of sexual excitement in some wild animals (e.g. deer, camel and elephant). In these animals spermatogenesis occurs only during this period.

2. Internal spermatic vein.
3. Vas deferens
4. Autonomic nerves from renal and caudal mesenteric plexus
5. Lymphatic vessels
6. Internal cremaster muscle
7. Tunica vaginalis propria.

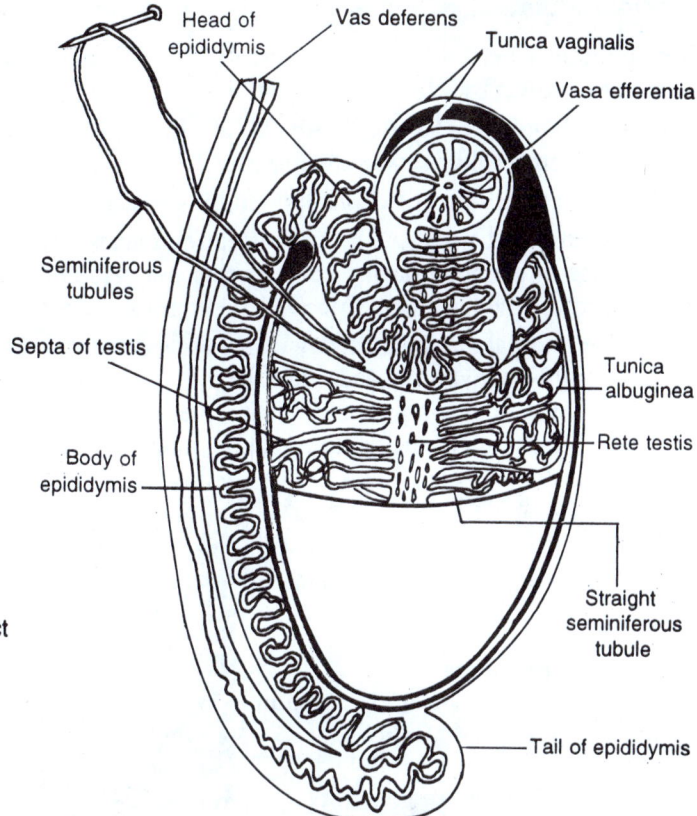

Fig. 1.4. Schematic diagram to show duct system of the testis and epididymis.

The **mesorchium** is delicate and double layer of peritoneum connecting visceral and parietal layer of vaginal process (as mesentery connects visceral and parietal layer of abdominal peritoneum) and continues up to dorsolateral abdominal wall.

In bull, ram and buck the testicles are placed in the scrotum vertically. In the stallion the testicles are placed nearly horizontally in the scrotum but when these are retracted, they become nearly vertical. In boar the long axis of the testis is oblique (neither vertical nor horizontal). Testicular details in different species are given in Table 1.1.

Table 1.1. Shape, colour of parenchyma and measurement of testis

	Horse	Bull	Ram	Boar	Dog	Cat
Shape	Oval	Elongated oval	Elongated oval	Elliptical	Round to oval	Round to oval
Parenchyma	Reddish gray	Yellow	Creamy white	Grayish to dark red	Reddish	Reddish
Measurement (cm)	$11 \times 6 \times 4$	$14 \times 7 \times 7$	$10 \times 6 \times 6$	$13 \times 7 \times 7$	1×1.2 to 4×2.5	1.2×0.7 to 2×1.5
Weight (gm)	200-300	250-300	200-300	150-200	7-15	—
Plane	Horizontal	Vertical	Vertical	Oblique	Oblique	Oblique

Thermoregulation of testes

For optimum production of the spermatozoa, the temperature of the testis be maintained at a temperature lower by 2 to 5°C than that of the body of the animal. This lowering of the temperature of testis is maintained by the following mechanisms.

1. The scrotal skin lacks subcutaneous fat.
2. The scrotal skin is richly supplied by sweat glands.
3. During cold weather, the cremaster and dartos muscles contract and thus testicles are held close to the body during cold. During hot weather, the cremaster and dartos muscles relax to lower the testis in a thin walled pendulous scrotum.
4. The internal spermatic artery enters the testis from the spermatic cord. The testicular artery is highly convoluted and cone shaped on the dorsal pole of the testis. These arterial coils are enmeshed with the pampiniform plexus of the testicular vein (Fig. 1.5). This arrangement further assists in the heat regulatory mechanisms of the testis. The arterial blood reaching the testis is cooled down by the venous blood leaving the testis.

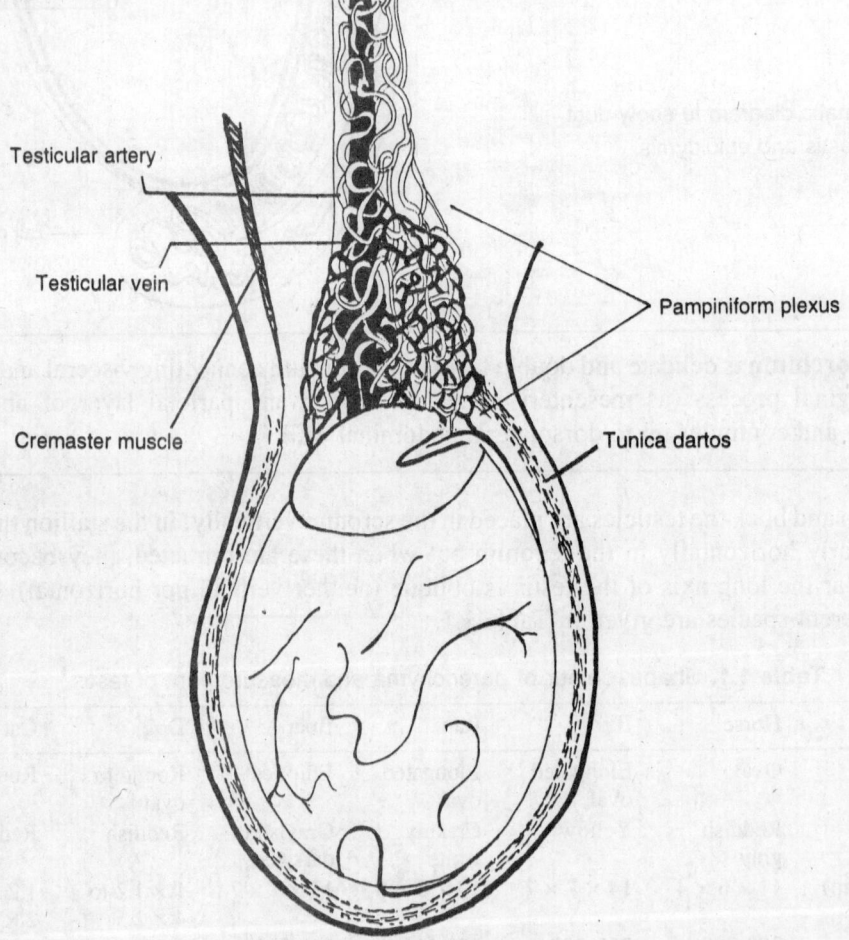

Fig. 1.5. Diagrammatic view to show pampiniform plexus and other structures that help in thermoregulation of testes in bull.

Functions of the testes

The following functions are performed by the testes :

1. Production of testosterone from the interstitial cells (Leydig's cells) lying between the seminiferous tubules (Endocrine function).
2. The spermatogonia situated peripherally in the seminiferous tubules undergo cell division and produce spermatozoa (Exocrine function). In bulls about 12-17 million spermatozoa are produced per gram of testicular tissue daily.

The above two important functional roles of the testes are controlled by the gonadotropic hormones of the pituitary. LH (ICSH) controls the endocrine activity of the Leydig's cells to produce testosterone. Testosterone produced by interstitial cells support the action of the FSH on spermatogenesis, develops and maintains the accessory sex glands, develops secondary sexual characteristics, develops sexual behaviour and is responsible for the functional maintenance of the male reproductive system. FSH controls spermatogenesis in the seminiferous tubules.

3. The blood testis barrier (at the level of the basement membrane of the seminiferous tubules and also by some special features of sustentacular cells) protect the germinal epithelium from the immunological damages.

EPIDIDYMIS

The epididymis is a coiled tube closely attached to the testis by fibrous tissue. The epididymis is more firm is consistency than the testis. The epididymis consists of head (caput), body (corpus) and tail (cauda). The length of the epididymal tube in different animals is :

Bull	30 m
Ram	50 m
Boar	50 m
Horse	20 m

The caput epididymis is broad, somewhat flat, U-shaped and covers nearly one third of the proximal end of the testis. The corpus epididymis is comparatively narrow part, running toward distal end of the testis along its posterior border. The cauda epididymis is enlarged end of the epididymis at the distal pole of the testis and is continuous with the vas deferens.

Histologically two prominent layers (1) circular muscle fibers layer and (2) pseudostratified columnar cells layer are seen in the epididymal wall. Based on histology, the epididymis can be divided in three segments (these segments do not coincide with the gross anatomical segments i.e. head, body and tail of the epididymis). The proximal segment has ciliated cells (having kinocilia) beating out-words. The lumen of the initial segment is almost obliterated (almost no lumen is present). The medusa formations seen in the semen ejaculates are actually the detached ciliated cells from this initial segment of the epididymis. In the middle segment of the epididymis, the lumen is wide and the cilia are not so straight. In the terminal segment of the epididymis the cilia are short, the lumen is very wide and is packed with spermatozoa.

Functions of the epididymis

Various functions of the epididymis are as follows :

1. Absorption

2. Secretion

3. Maturation

4. Transportation and

5. Storage

Absorption : The fluid released by testes is several times more than the volume of the semen ejaculate. It is estimated that ram's testes produce about 60 ml fluid daily while only about 1 ml semen ejaculate is obtained. The epithelial cells of the epididymis, especially of the tail region are involved in the active absorption of fluid. Thus in the cauda epididymis the spermatozoa suspension is highly concentrated.

Secretion : The secretions of the epididymal cells maintain viability of the spermatozoa during storage.

Maturation : During the storage period in the epididymis, the spermatozoa undergo maturation changes. There is migration of the cytoplasmic droplet from the neck of the spermatozoa (proximal protoplasmic droplet) to the distal end of the middle piece (distal protoplasmic droplet) in bull. This change is associated with cytochemical changes in the spermatozoa leading to its increased capacity for motility and fertilizing ability.

Transportation : The transportation of the spermatozoa from rete testis to the efferent tubules is mainly due to the presence of testicular fluid. The further transport of the spermatozoa is due to action of the ciliated epithelium and the action of peristaltic waves of the muscle fibers in the duct. The average duration of the epididymal journey of the spermatozoa in different species is :

Bull	10 days
Ram	13-15 days
Boar	9-12 days
Stallion	8-11 days

Storage : The epididymis is the store house for spermatozoa. The two epididymides in bull can accommodate up to 3-4 days production of spermatozoa by the testis (nearly up to 75×10^9 spermatozoa). The cauda epididymis stores nearly 50% of the extragonadal sperms. However, sperms in the epididymis remain in quiescent metabolic state.

VAS DEFERENS

The two ductus deferens or vas deferens extend from cauda epididymis to the pelvic urethra. The ducts are firm with thick muscular walls and lumen quite small. The ducts are convoluted near the cauda epididymis and then run parallel to the corpus epididymis. Later, these pass through the inguinal canal into the abdominal cavity along with other components of the spermatic card. On reaching the abdominal cavity, the vas deferens separates from the spermatic card, passes upward and backward to open into the pelvic urethra. The vas deferens is about 3 mm thick in bull and about 6 mm thick in stallion. The terminal part of the vas deferens is enlarged and is called ampulla. The ampulla is furnished with branched tubular glands. The ampulla in bulls measures about 10 to 12 cm in length and 1.0 to 1.5 cm in diameter. *There are no ampullae in dog and cat.* The ampullae open in the cranial portion of the pelvic urethra through a rounded prominence called **"colliculus seminalis"**. In the vas deferens the sperm transport is due to peristaltic waves.

ACCESSORY SEX GLANDS

1. The vesicular glands (Seminal vesicles)

The vesicular glands of the bull are paired accessory sex glands having distinct lobulations. These glands are located on the pelvic floor cranial and lateral to the ampullae. Branched tubular secretory glands present in the vascular glands add volume, nutrition and buffers in the semen. These glands open in the pelvic urethra near the opening of the ampullae (colliculus seminalis) or the duct of the vesicular gland and the ampulla may share a common ejaculatory orifice into the pelvic urethra. The approximate dimensions of the vesicular glands in different species are as follows :

	Length (cm)	Breadth (cm)	Thickness (cm)	Weight (gm)
Bull	10-15	2.0-4.0	2.0	75.0
Stallion	15-20	2.5-5.0	5.0	—
Boar	12-15	5.0-8.0	4.0	200.0
Ram	4-5	2.0	1.5	5.0

The secretions of the vesicular glands make up about 50% of the total semen ejaculate. Compared to prostatic secretions, the vesicular secretions are more alkaline. The secretion contains protein, fructose, ascorbic acid, citric acid, potassium bicarbonate, acid soluble phosphate and several enzymes. In mammals most of the seminal fructose comes from vesicular glands. The vesicular glands of the stallion are elongated pear shaped sacs and the secretions of these glands constitute gel to the ejaculate. In boar the vesicular glands are large bag like and contains a milky and highly viscous fluid. In boar the vesicular secretion has high inositol contents and also contains ergothioneine. In bulls the secretion of vesicular gland is yellow due to high riboflavin contents. *These glands are absent in dog and cat.*

2. The prostate gland

The prostate gland has different forms in different species. In bull the gland is located on the pelvic floor, on or around the neck of the bladder or the cranial portion of the pelvic urethra. The gland opens into the pelvic urethra lateral to the "colliculus seminalis" (opening of the ampullae) through many ducts. In dog there are only two excretory ducts of prostate gland.

In bull the prostrate gland surrounds the pelvic urethra and has two parts, the body of the prostate (pars propria) and the pars disseminata which surrounds the pelvic urethra. The approximate dimensions of the prostate gland in bull and boar are as follows :

	Pars propria (cm)	Pars disseminata (cm)
Bull	$3 \times 1 \times 1$	$12 \times 1.5 \times 1.0$
Boar	$3 \times 3 \times 1$	$17 \times 1.0 \times 1.0$

In ram, the prostate gland has no body and is scattered over the large portion of the pelvic urethra. In stallion, the prostate gland consists of two lateral lobes (each $7 \times 4 \times 1$ cm) connected by isthmus ($2 \times 3 \times 0.5$ cm).

In dog the size of the prostate gland varies greatly and may be quite large in older dogs. Some disseminate lobes are present in the urethral wall.

The prostatic secretions are rich in enzymes that resemble interior milieu of the cells rather than the external milieu of the cells e.g. glycolitic enzymes, proteinases, phosphatases, glycosidases, nucleases and nucleotidases. In dog the pH of the prostatic secretion is 6.5 and there are no reducing sugars. However, canine prostate secretion contains citric acid and acid phosphatase. Canine prostate secretion has high concentration of zinc. Zinc concentration in the seminal plasma is chiefly due to prostatic secretion.

3. The bulbourethral glands (Cowper's glands)

In bull, the bulbourethral glands are the paired glands lying on either side of the pelvic urethra in the region near the ischial arch. In bull, these glands are embedded under the bulbospongiosus muscle. These gland are ovoid in bull, stallion and ram and are large and cylindrical in boar. *These glands are absent in dog.* In cat these are of the size of the prostate. The dimensions of the bulbouretheral gland in different species of animals are as follows :

	Diameter (cm)	Length (cm)
Bull	1.5-3.0	—
Stallion	2.5-5.0	—
Ram	0.5-1.0	—
Boar	2.5-3.0	12.0

In bull and boar each gland opens in urethra through a single duct, but in stallion each gland opens into the urethra through 6 to 8 secretary ducts. In bulls, the dribbling seen from the prepuce prior to mounting are secretions from the prostate and bulbourethral glands. These secretions delete harmful substances if present in the urethra and clean it prior to semen ejaculation. The typical rubber like white substance is filled in the Cowper's glands of the boar that is essential for gel formation in boar semen.

URETHRA

The urethra in males is the common passage for the excretion of urine as well as for the transportation of semen. The urethra has three distinct parts (pelvic part, bulb of urethra and the penile part). In bull, the pelvic part of urethra is about 20 cm in length and is situated on pelvic floor. The pelvic urethra is enclosed by heavy urethral muscle. The bulb of urethra is extra pelvic part situated at ischial arch and is bending ventral to the pelvis. The penile urethra runs inside the penis proper. **Urethral glands** are seen in man. These gland are absent in bull and stallion. However in boar, urethral glands are distinct.

PENIS

The penis is the copulatory organ in males. The penile body is largely composed of corpus cavernosum penis. The corpus cavernosum penis arises as a pair of crura or roots from the ischial arch under ischiocavernosus muscle. The carpus cavernosum penis is enclosed by a thick layer of tunica albuginea, which is made up of collagen fibres. Several trabeculae are sent from tunica albuginea to enter into the corpus cavernosum penis for the support of cavernous (cave like) tissue. Ventral to the corpus cavernosum penis and surrounding the penile urethra is smaller corpus spongiosum penis (also called corpus spongiosum urethrae) as shown in Fig. 1.6. The carpus

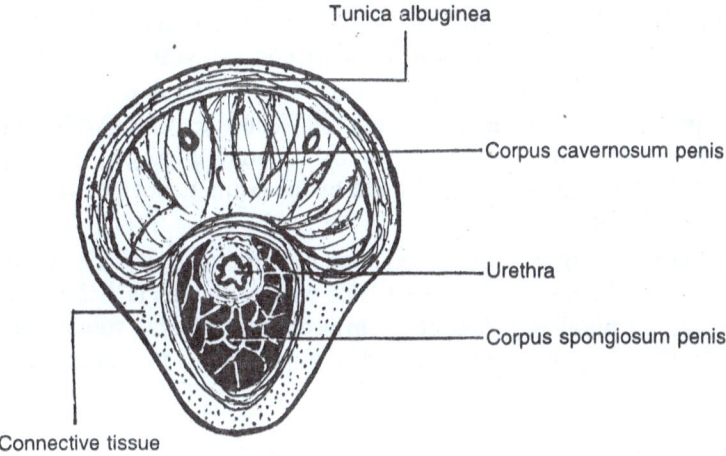

Fig. 1.6. Schematic diagram of the cross section of the penis of bull near caudal end.

spongiosum penis in enlarged at ischial arch to form the penile bulb. The bulb is covered by bulbospongiosus muscle (also called bulbocavernosus muscle). The two corpora (corpus cavernosum penis and corpus spongiosum penis) have several spaces (blood sinusoids) regarded as enlarged capillaries and are continuous with veins in the penis. Distention of these spaces with blood, causes penile erection. In bull, ram, and boar the penis is characterized by S-shaped curve, the sigmoid flexure. The sigmoid flexure is post-scrotal in bull and ram and pre-scrotal in boar. Sigmoid flexure is absent in horse. Inchiocavernosus muscle or erector penis muscle is a short paired muscle and helps penile erection by its compressing and pumping action. The retractor penis muscle is a smooth muscle and arises from sacral or first and second coccigeal regions, divides and meets again under the anus and attaches to the penis at the distal end of the sigmoid flexure with fibers extending dorsally on the penis. The thickened dorsal portion of this fibrous sheath is known as dorsal apical ligament of the penis. The retractor penis muscle draws the penis back into sheath by acting on sigmoid flexure.

The penis of the **bull** is about 90 cm in length from its root to the tip of the glans. The diameter is about 4 to 5 cm on erection. The glans penis is 7.5 to 12.5 cm long and is rather pointed. The glans penis (terminal part) is pointed and slightly twisted. After intromission the spirally arranged fibrous penile and prepenile prepuce is stretched and this causes the penis to spiral (Fig. 1.7). The penis of the bull is fibroelastic and the erectile tissue is too less compared to stallions.

The penis of the **stallion** has large amount of the erectile tissue. The length is about 50 cm and the diameter about 2.5 to 6.0 cm when not erect. A length of about 15 to 20 cm lies free in the prepuce. The length of the penis increases to about double and of the glans penis to about triple on erection. There is a prominent urethral process in the glans penis (Fig. 1.7) encircled by a shallow groove called as fossa glandis which forms urethral sinus or diverticulum, dorsal to the urethral process. The diverticulum (sinus) is often filled with smegma and carries infection, causing contagious equine metritis. The retractor penis muscle is not as strong as in bulls.

T' ₌ penis of the **ram** is about 30 cm in length and 1.5 to 2.0 cm in diameter and is characterized by urethral process, which extends 4 to 5 cm beyond the glans penis (Fig. 1.7).

The penile length of the **boar** is about 45 to 55 cm. There is no glans penis but the cranial portion is twisted counter clockwise (Fig. 1.7).

The penile length of **dog** during non-erect condition varies from about 6.5 to 24 cm depending upon the size of the dog. The penis of dog has two separate corpora cavernosa (separated by a medial septum). The cranial free portion of the penis contains a bone called "os penis" which is grooved ventrally for urethral passage. The glans penis of the dog consists of two parts. The proximal one third part of the glans is "bulbus glandis" and the distal two third part is "pars longa glandis". The proximal part "bulbus glandis" usually becomes engorged with blood after the penis enters the vagina of the bitch and the withdrawal of the penis is not possible for some time after service until erection subsides.

The penis of the **cat** is short and is directed caudally and ventrally. The urethra lies dorsally in the penis. The os penis is either absent or short. The bulbus glandis is also absent. The glans penis is also absent but the terminal part (about 1 cm) contains several spines (about 120) pointing backward (Fig. 1.7). Because of the pain caused by these spines the queen emits a loud cry after service.

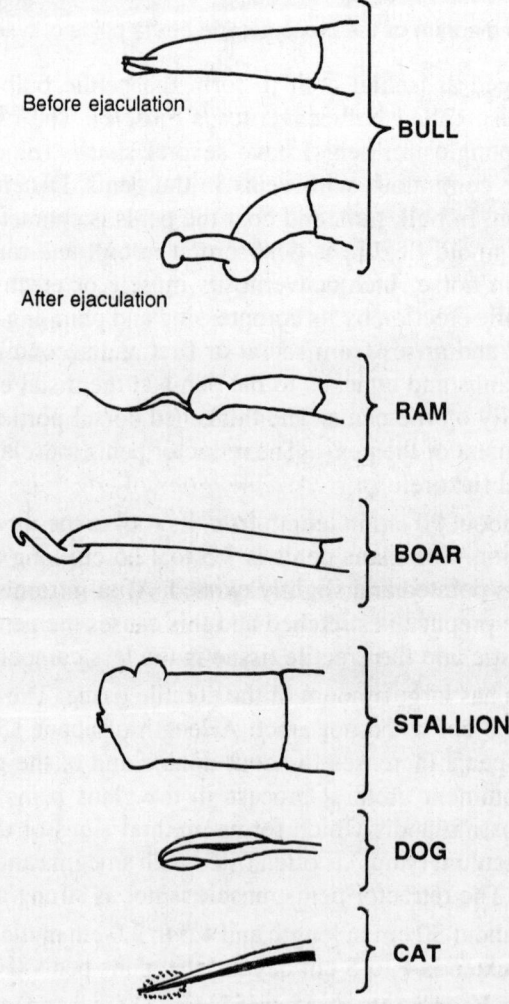

Before ejaculation

BULL

After ejaculation

RAM

BOAR

STALLION

DOG

CAT

Fig. 1.7. Diagrams showing free end of penis in bull, ram, boar, stallion, dog and cat.

PREPUCE

The prepuce is the invaginated fold of skin surrounding the free end of the penis, when not erect.

- The prepuce in the **bull** is about 35 cm long and 4 cm in diameter. The prepucial orifice is 5 to 7 cm behind umbilicus and is surrounded by tuft of hair. In the bulls of Indian breeds, the prepuce is in the form of pendulous sheath.
- The prepuce of the **horse** makes a double fold. The prepucial cavity is 15 to 20 cm deep and then there is second fold to form the prepuce proper. Prepucial ring is prominent in between the two prepucial folds.
- The prepuce of **ram** is similar to bull but is relatively short.
- The prepuce of **boar** has a diverticulum (pouch) dorsal to the prepucial orifice. This diverticulum is filled with urine, secretions and dead cells and thus produces typical odour.

BLOOD AND NERVE SUPPLY

The **testicle** is supplied blood from internal spermatic artery originating directly from aorta. The internal spermatic veins run parallel to the internal spermatic artery except near testis where it is more convoluted and tortuous to form pampiniform plexus, which plays important role in the thermoregulation of the testes. The nerve supply to the testis is through fibers from renal and caudal mesenteric plexus. These fibers run close to the internal spermatic artery.

The blood to the **scrotum** is supplied by the external pudendal artery (also the internal pudendal artery in cat and boar). The nerve supply to the scrotum is by genital nerve (which is a branch of genito-femoral nerve arising from second to fourth lumber nerves and perineal nerve).

The blood supply to the **penis** is through internal pudendal artery (to the root of the penis, obturator artery (to the body of the penis) and the external pudendal artery which gives rise to dorsal artery of the penis after passing through the inguinal canal. The nerve supply to the penis is from autonomic nerves from pelvic plexus and from pudendal and hemorrhoidal nerves. The pudendal and hemorrhoidal nerves are the motor nerves for retractor penis muscles. The dorsal nerve of the penis is a branch of pudendal nerve and supplies sensory fibers to the glans penis. These sensory fibers provide the afferent side for the reflex of erection and ejaculation. The reflex centers for erection and ejaculation are located in the lumber portion of the spinal cord.

The blood supply to the **accessory sex gland** in large animal is from internal pudendal artery. In dog the supply to accessory sex glands is from prostatic artery (a branch of urogenital artery arising from internal iliac artery). The nerve supply to the accessory sex glands is through autonomic nerves from hypogastric nerve and pelvic plexus.

Chapter 2

The Embryology of the Male Reproductive Tract

In the early embryonic life nephric and genital regions are formed from the mesodermal tissue and these regions finally develop into the urogenital system. The segmental tubules in the cranial portion of the nephric region form pronephros, each with a pronephric duct that runs to primitive cloaca. Later on, caudal to prenephros other segmental tubules form another temporary excretory organ, the mesonephros (Wolffian body) and mesonephric ducts (Wolffian ducts) that unite with the pronephric ducts. The prenephros degenerates. Later on, from the out growth of the meso-nephric duct (Wolffian duct) a third and more permanent excretory organ develop more caudally to form metanephros or true kidney with its ureter and bladder (Fig. 2.1). The mesonephros (Wolffian body) also degenerates but the mesonephric duct is utilized in males for spermatozoa transport from testis to pelvic urethra.

Initially the site of the gonad is microscopically visible in the genital region on the medial side of the middle part of each mesonephros as gonadal ridge or genital ridge, which is aggregation of mesodermal cells located between the dorsal mesentery and the mesonephros. The sex of the embryo is finalized at fertilization but during the early stage of embryonic development it remains very difficult, if not impossible, to differentiate male and female embryos and this stage is referred to as **"indifferent stage"**. As long as prospective testis and ovary remain indistinguishable it is referred to as gonad. Gender specific characteristics develop shortly there after accompanied by degeneration of inappropriate structures. The differentiation of the gonads occurs both during the prenatal and post-natal periods. The prenatal differentiation seems to be under inherent genetic potential and the postnatal differentiation under circulating hormonal levels. The genital ridge is formed when the embryo is about 24 days in canine and ovine, 27 days in equine and 28 days in bovine. It is an interesting fact that primary germ cells are not derived from the gonadal precursors. The origin of the primary germ cells is extra gonadal, from the wall of yolk sac endoderm in the region of hind gut. These primordial germ cells from the wall of the yolk sac shift dorsally to occupy the dorsal mesentery of the hind gut and then to the medial side of middle part of the each mesonephros, which is the site of the genital, ridge formation (Fig. 2.2).

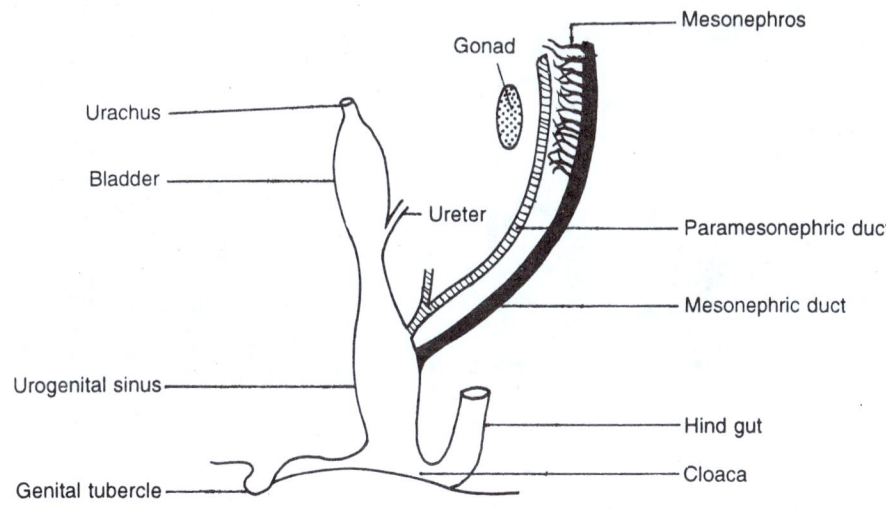

Fig. 2.1. Schematic diagram to show urogenital system at indifferent stage.

GONADOGENESIS IN MALES

The indifferent stage : Cords of the epithelial cells from mesonephric tubules and degenerating glomerular capsule invade the area of the gonadal ridge. These cords coalesce (Grow into each other) to form clusters and small vesicles that incorporate primary germ cells (Fig. 2.3 A & B). These cords of epithelial components are called gonadal cords (primitive sex cords). These primitive sex cords establish a epithelial network between gonadal ridge epithelium and the remnants of the mesonephric tubules. Up to this stage the gonad is indifferent

   Testis : The gonadal cords are made up of primitive germ cells and the supporting Sertoli cells (sustentacular cells) and are solid tubes that becomes patent (evident) postnatally and form semeniferous tubules (Fig. 2.3 D & F). Seminiferous tubules remain solid until just before puberty. These tubules are connected to efferent ductules via a network of ductules called rete testis. The pri-

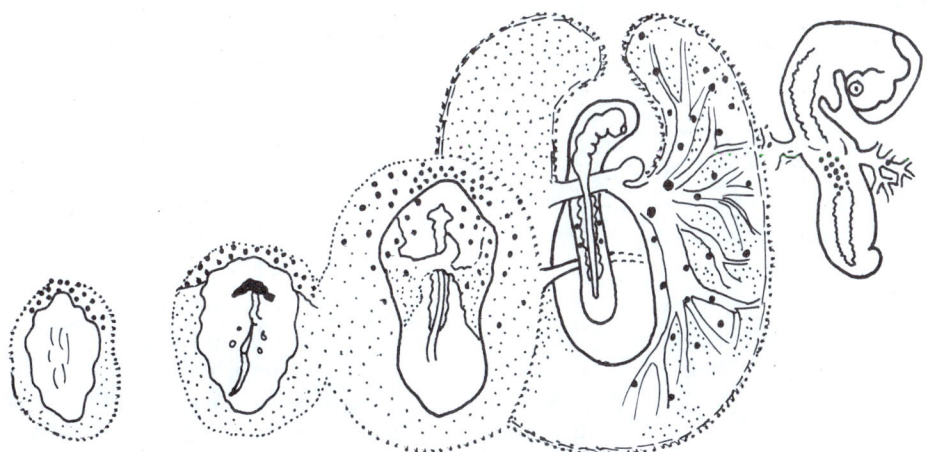

Fig. 2.2. Schematic diagrams to show that primordial germ cells (bigger black spots) appear in the wall of yolk sac endoderm and then through circulation reach the genital ridge.

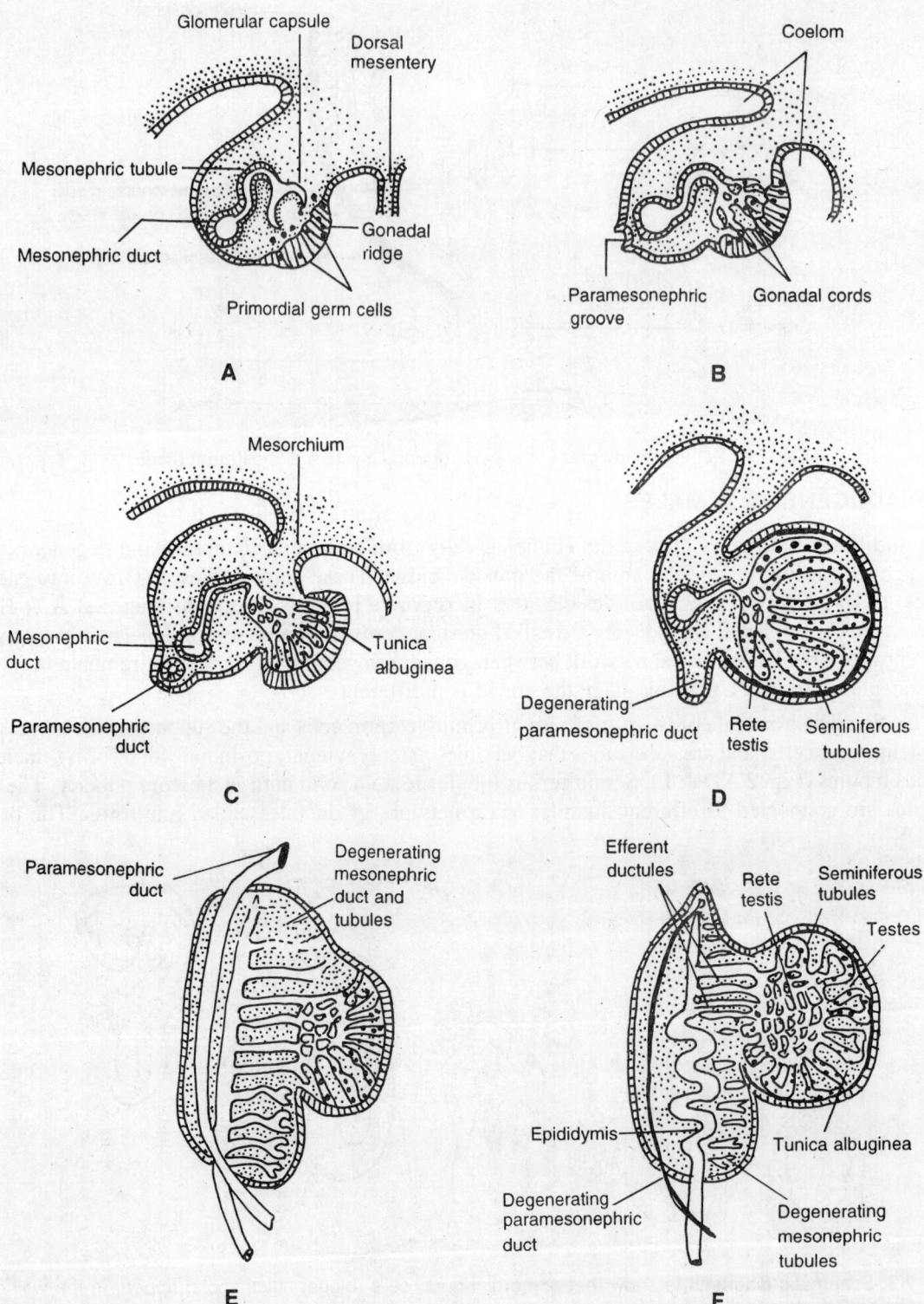

Fig. 2.3. Schematic diagram to show development of testis. A & B are indifferent stages. A, B, C & D are transverse views. E & F are the ventral views of the C & D stages, respectively.

mordial tunica albuginea (a distinct mesenchymal sheet) develops and separates gonadal cords from the coelomic epithelium (Fig. 2.3 C). Initial appearance of the tunica albuginea in the first histological evidence denoting onset of testicular development. It takes several day for tunica albuginea to fully encapsulate the testis. The Sertoli cells (sustentacular cells) are derived from ' mesonephric tubule epithelial cells. The origin of the interstitial cells (Leydig cells) located between seminiferous tubules is rather uncertain, but it is believed that interstitial cells are formed by mesodermal mesenchyme cells that originally occupied the gonadal ridge.

Ovary : In females epithelial gonadal cords break up to form many small clusters called follicles each containing one or more germ cells in the centre. Most of these follicles are located peripherally towards the hypertrophied epithelium that would form mesothelial surface of the ovary. The follicles situated in the deep medullary region degenerate and blood vessels develop in the medullary region. The mare is an exception in which the follicles are distributed throughout the ovary (not in the cortical region only) and the vascular supply is peripheral. Tunica albuginea does not develop in the ovary. (Tunica albuginea is the first histological evidence that the developing gonad is a testis). Most of the oogonia divide mitotically during fetal stage and shortly after birth. When they stop dividing they form primary oocytes (Fig. 2.4).

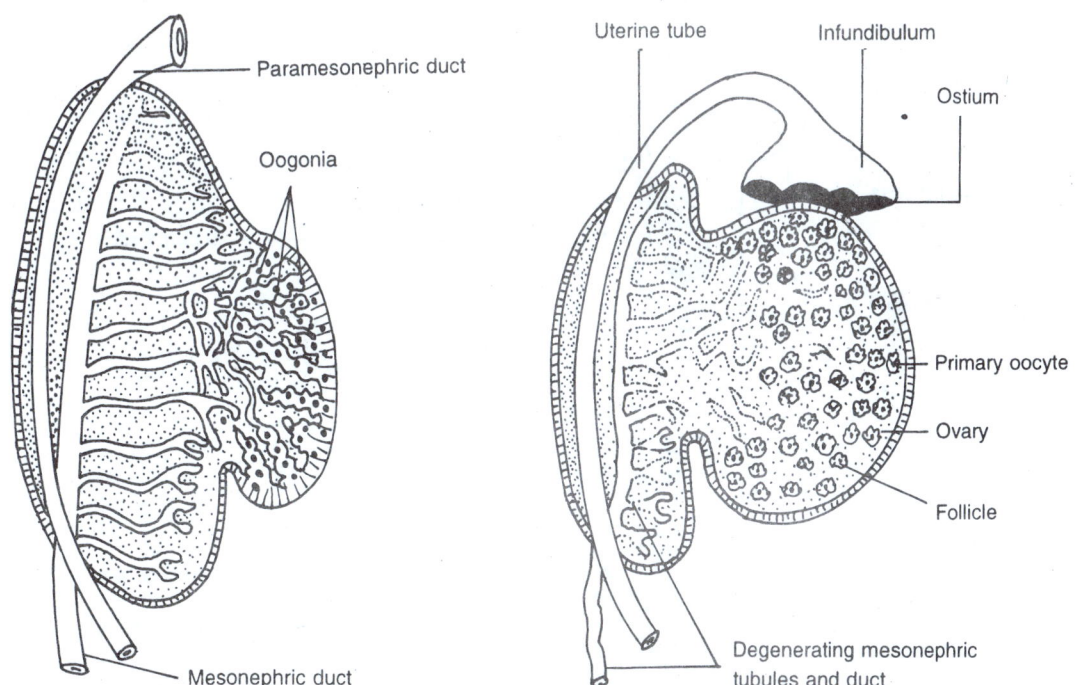

Fig. 2.4. Schematic diagrams to show development of ovary (ventral views).

DESCENT OF THE TESTICLE

In the females, the ovaries remain in the abdominal cavity fairly close to the place of their origin, but in males the testes travel a considerable distance from their point of origin (near the caudal pole of the kidney) and sink through inguinal canal into the scrotum (Fig. 2.5). The testicular descent is preceded by the formation of the vaginal process, which is a peritoneal sac extending ɔwards scrotum and enclosing the inguinal ligament of the testis. The inguinal ligament connects

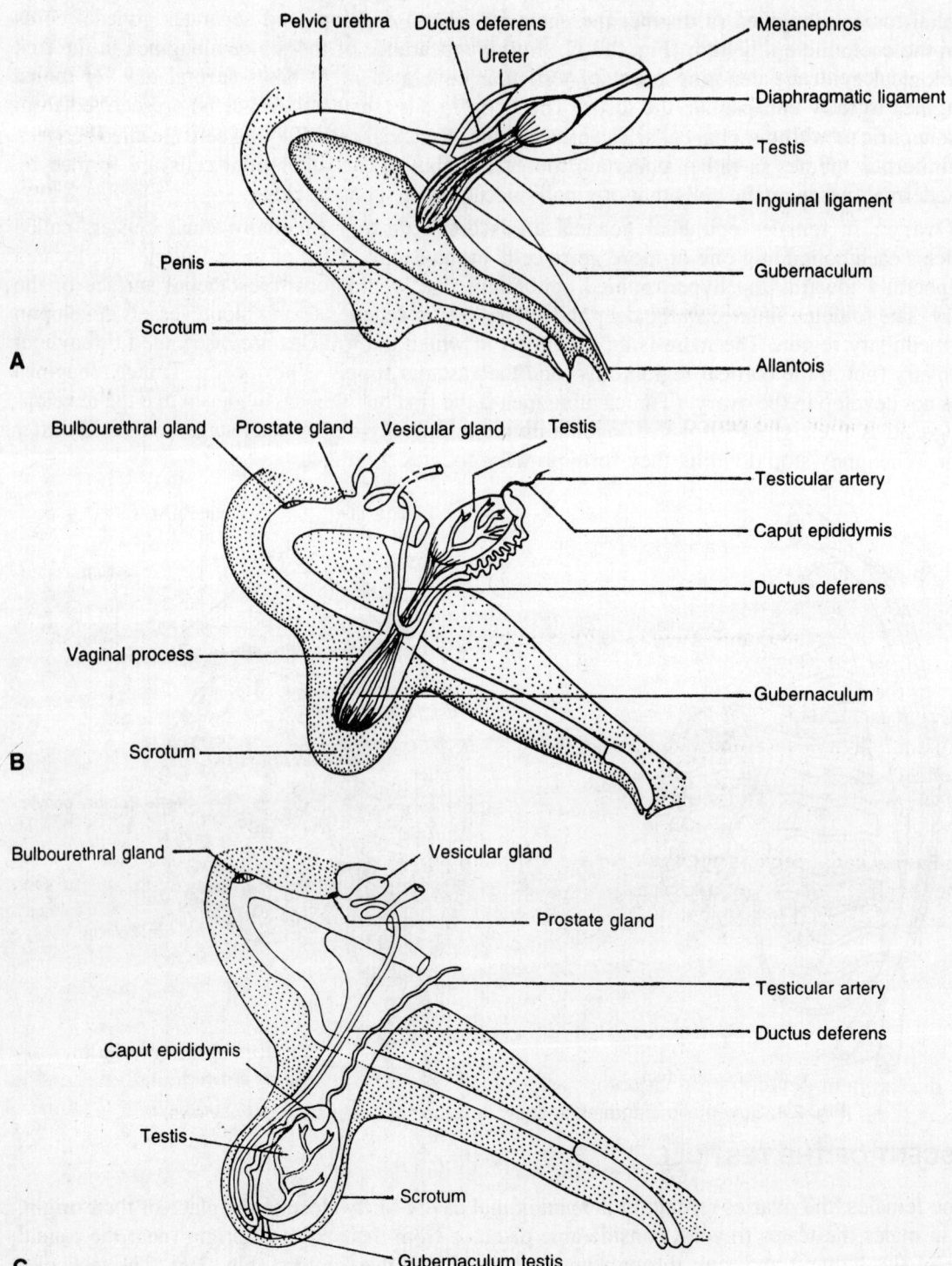

Fig. 2.5. Schematic diagrams to show testicular descent (A to C) and development of reproductive tract in bovine foetus.

the gonad and the mesonephric duct. The inguinal ligament together with diaphragmatic ligament and mesorchium suspends the testes of the fetus. The testicles covered by the visceral peritoneum moves caudoventrally guided by gubernaculum, which is fibrous mesenchymal cord extending from labio-scrotal swelling to the gonad. As a result of cell proliferation and increase in the secretion of extracellular matrix material consisting mostly of hyaluronic acid, the gubernaculum swells at the level of the inguinal canal. The accumulation of this extracellular secretion dilates the inguinal canal and also makes the gubernaculum more soft and jelly like in consistency and thus the resistance for testicular descent in decreased. The process of testicular descent is passive. There is no contractile tissue present in the gubernaculum to actively pull the gonad through the inguinal canal. The testis governs its own descent. The testicular descent is probably hormonally controlled by androgens from testes or adrenals. The gubernacular out growth is stimulated by non-androgenic testicular factors that are enhanced by testosterone. After the descent of testes, through the inguinal canal into the scrotum, the gubernaculum regresses and decreases in size. The gubernaculum forms the ligamentum testis and the scrotal ligament. The descent of testicles in normally completed by birth or soon after. The period of testicular descent through inguinal canal in different species is as follows :

Bull	106 days of gestation
Ram	70 days of gestation
Boar	70 days of gestation
Horse	at or near birth
Dog	3-4 days postnatally; however, the canine testes reach the scrotal location by about a month after birth

Cryptorchidism is the condition in which one or both the testes are retained either in the abdominal cavity or in the inguinal canal. The animal in which the testicle descends in to the inguinal canal but not into the scrotum is called **"high flanker"**. A cryptorchid with both the testes retained in the abdominal cavity is very likely to be sterile. For normal spermatogenesis a relatively cooler temperature (than the body temperature) is required which is met only in scrotum. Normally the inguinal canal permits passage only for spermatic cord along with inguinal vessels and nerves. If the inguinal canal is too relaxed, it may allow to pass loop of intestine into the scrotum and thus producing **inguinal hernia**.

THE ORIGIN OF THE INTERNAL DUCTS

During the early embryonic stage, all the vertebrate embryos have a double set of sex ducts and both the sex ducts are held intact during the indifferent period. Later during differentiation only one duct system develops and the other regresses. Each sex whether male or female carries the organs of the opposite sex as rudiments but these remnant rudiments do not interfere in the normal functioning of the prevailing sex system.

The mesonephric tubules and the mesonephric ducts (Wolffian ducts) are used very extensively by the male for the permanent duct system and the paramesonephric ducts (mullerian ducts) become rudimentary (Fig. 2.6). In females, it is just reverse. The mesonephros degenerate from cranial to caudal. In males some of the mesonephric tubules that fuse with gonadal cords persist and form the efferent ductules. The portion of the mesonephric duct (Wolffian duct) closely associated with the testis forms epididymis. The caudal part of the mesonephric duct forms ductus deferens (Vas

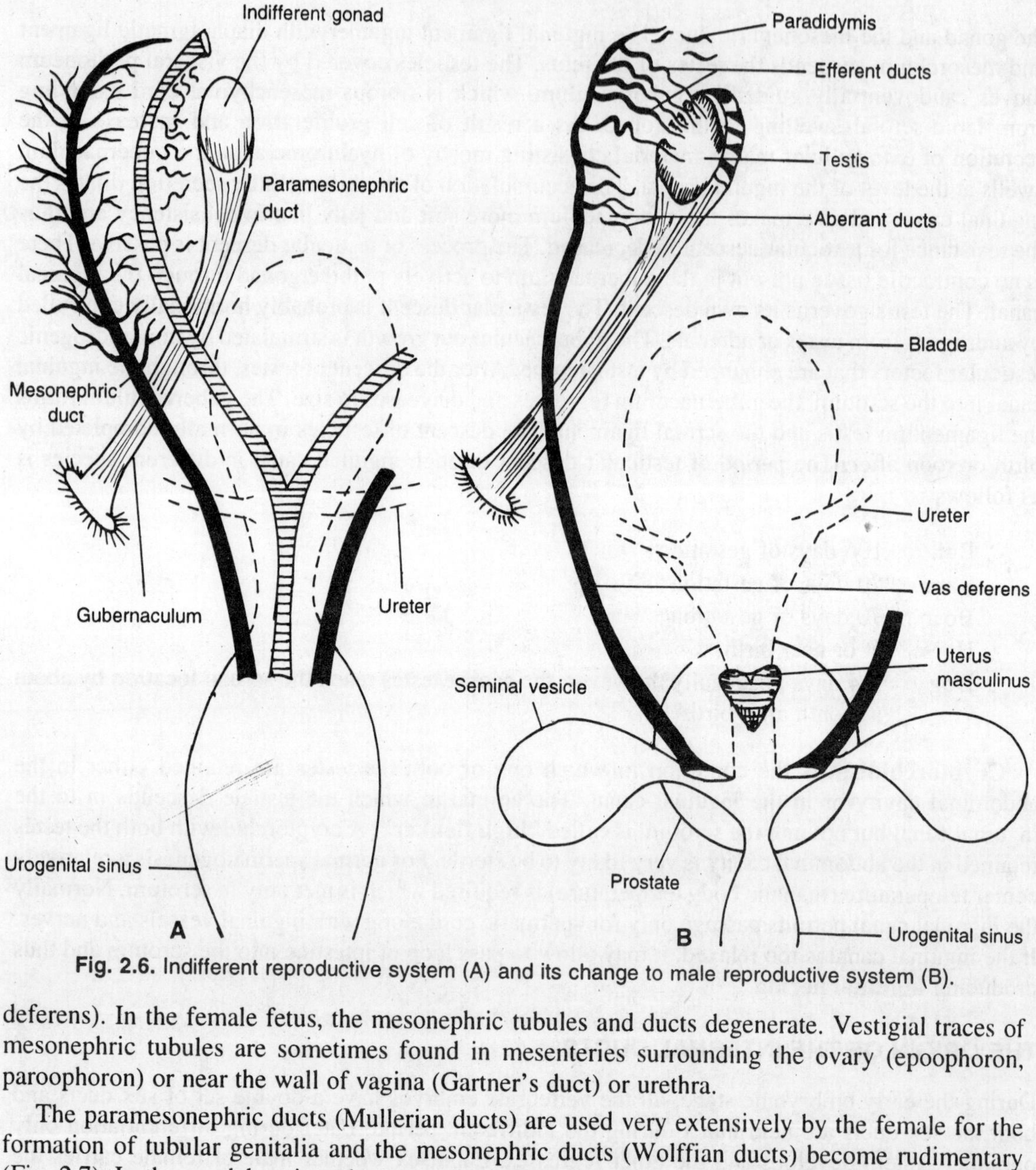

Fig. 2.6. Indifferent reproductive system (A) and its change to male reproductive system (B).

deferens). In the female fetus, the mesonephric tubules and ducts degenerate. Vestigial traces of mesonephric tubules are sometimes found in mesenteries surrounding the ovary (epoophoron, paroophoron) or near the wall of vagina (Gartner's duct) or urethra.

The paramesonephric ducts (Mullerian ducts) are used very extensively by the female for the formation of tubular genitalia and the mesonephric ducts (Wolffian ducts) become rudimentary (Fig. 2.7). In the caudal region, the paramesonephric ducts unite and extend caudally as one tube to enter the urogenital sinus. The cranial portion of the paramesonephric duct (mullerian duct) develops in female to form the oviduct while the caudal portion fuse in varying degree and develop to form the uterine horn, uterine body, cervix and nearly cranial two-third or more of vagina. The rest of the portion of the vagina is formed by the urogenital sinus. The caudal part of the urogenital sinus is retained as vestibule. In the male fetus, the paramesonephric ducts degenerate. Vestigial traces of the paramesonephric ducts include appendix of testis (cranially) and uterus masculinus (caudally).

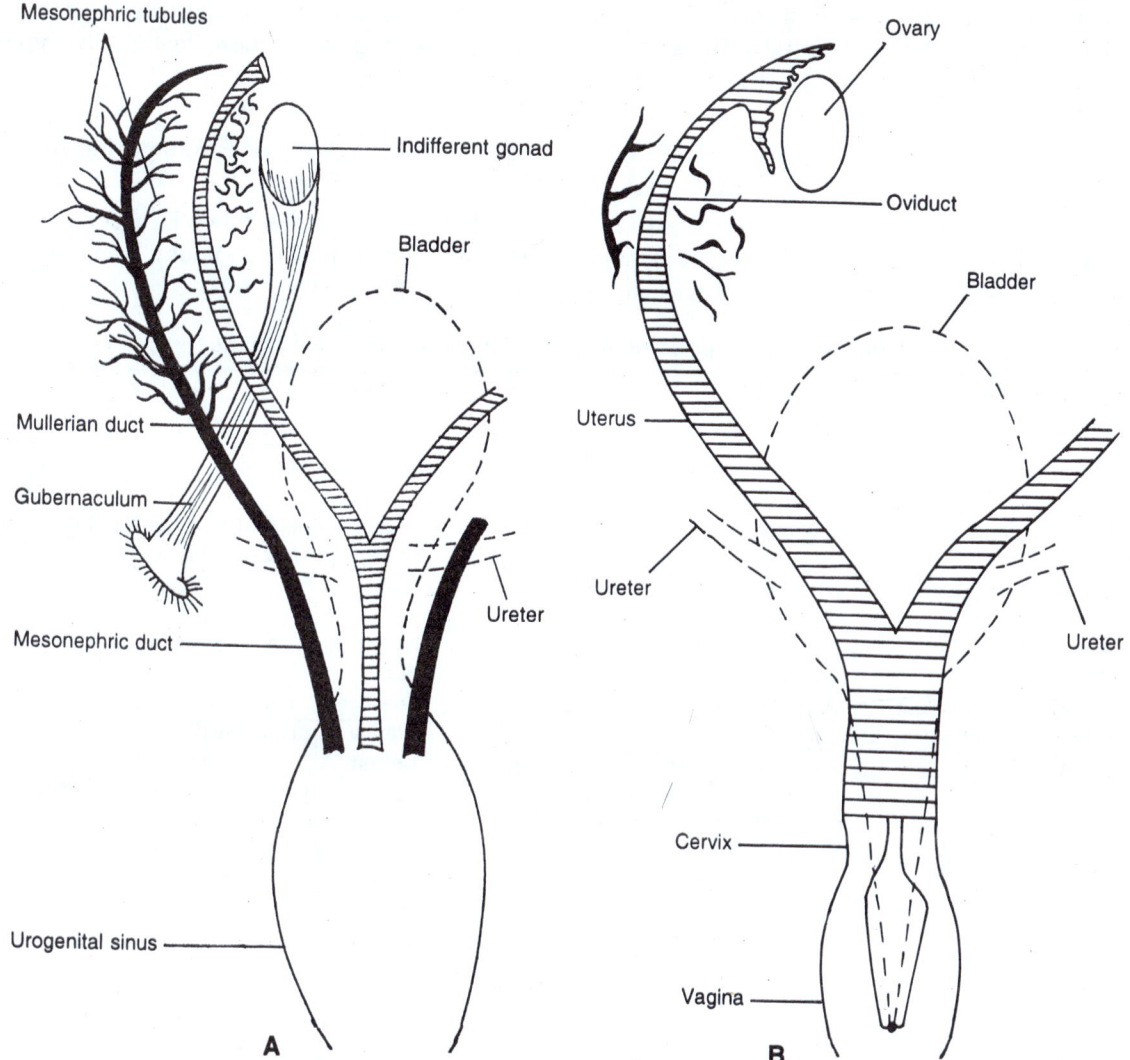

Fig. 2.7. Indifferent reproductive system (A) and its change to female reproductive system (B).

ORIGIN OF THE ACCESSORY SEX GLANDS

The prostate and bulbourethral glands (Cowper's glands) develop as out growth from the epithelium of the urogenital sinus. The seminal vesicles develop from mesonephric ducts (Wolffian ducts).

The cat lacks seminal vesicles and the dog has only a prostate gland.

ORIGIN OF THE EXTERNAL GENITALIA

The external genitalia also develops from an indifferent stage possessing all the rudimentary anatomical features of both the sexes. Proliferation of the mesoderm adjacent to the cloacal membrane creates a series of swelling. Later, at the cranial end develops genital tubercle and at the caudal end develops genital folds. As the development progresses, these features become accentuated as per the sex-genetic picture of the embryo.

If the embryo is genetically destined to develop as male, the genital tubercle enlarges to become the penis. The penis is partially enclosed by the prepuce, which is developed from genital folds. The scrotal pouches are derived from genital swellings.

If the embryo is genetically destined to become a female, the genital tubercle becomes the clitoris. The genital swellings make labia majora and genital folds make labia minora. Homologies of male and female reproductive organs are given in Table 1.2.

Table 1.2. Homologies of male and female reproductive organs

Indifferent embryonic structure	Adult male	Adult female
Gonad	Testis, rete testis	Ovary, rete ovarii*
Mesentery	Mesorchium	Mesovarium
Gubernaculum	Ligamentum testis	Round ligament of the uterus and the proper ligament of the ovary
Mesonephric tubules	Efferent ducts, Paradidymis*, Vas aberrans*	Epoohoron*, Paroophoron*
Mesonephric duct (Wolffian duct)	Epididymis, Vas deferens, Seminal vesicle	Duct-part of Epoophoron* (Gartner's duct)
Paramesonephric duct (Mullerian duct)	Appendage of testis*, Uterus masculinus*	Oviducts, Uterus, Cervix, Vagina (Cranial portion)
Urogenital sinus	Prostalic, membranous and cavernous urethra; Bulbourethral glands (Cowper's glands); Prostate	Urethra, Vestibule, Vagina (Caudal part), Vestibular glands (Bartholin's glands), Paraurethral glands*
Genital swelling	Scrotal pouch	Labia majora
Genital tubercle	Penis	Clitoris
Genital fold	Prepuce	Labia minora

* Rudimentary

Chapter 3

Growth, Puberty, Sexual Maturity and Libido

The development of the reproductive organs is comparatively slow before puberty. The puberty is defined as the period when the sexual organs are functionally developed, the innate sexual interests are prominent, the animal is able to produce spermatozoa and is able to copulate resulting in pregnancy in females. Other definitions of puberty are also cited in literature and one definition commonly associated to bulls is "the age at which the first ejaculate contains 50×10^6 (50 million) sperms with at least 10% progressive motility". Puberty is the result of the adjustment of testes to respond to the effect of gonadotropins from the anterior pituitary for steriodogenesis and gametogenesis. The puberty does not denote the full reproductive capacity, which is achieved later, on attaining maturity. Maturity occurs when physiological, including spermatogenic developments and behavioural developments are fully co-ordinated to allow fertile service to occur. After puberty, there is increase in the ejaculate volume, increase in the percentage of the motile spermatozoa in semen, increase in the sperm concentration in the ejaculate and decrease in the number of spermatozoa with proximal protoplasmic droplets. In cattle bull, the volume of the ejaculate increases up to nearly 6 years of age and in buffalo bulls, it increases up to nearly 7 years of age. The physiological growth of the body in more important for the onset of puberty than the age of the animal. The onset of puberty is a gradual process and occurs after achieving optimum body weight, which is influenced by plane of nutrition, management practices, breed of the animal, cross-breeding, disease conditions and individual differences. The age at puberty in males of different species is :

Bull	1.0-1.5 years (Exotic breeds)
	1.5-2.0 years (Zebu breeds)
Buffalo	2.0-2.5 years
Stallion	1.5 years
Ram	7-8 months
Boar	6-7 months
Dog	8-10 months
Cat	9-10 months

The puberty in males is brought about by the maturation of the pituitary gland and the release of gonadotropins from it. The gonadotropins from the anterior pituitary brings about maturation of the gonads which in turn secrete steroid hormones. The steroid hormones from the gonads cause development of the genital organs and the secondary sex characteristics. Thus the onset of puberty is controlled by the interaction of the anterior pituitary and the gonads. The secretion of STH and FSH is continual from the anterior pituitary even from the prenatal life but he FSH is released in sufficient functional amount later in post-natal life. FSH from the anterior pituitary gland initiates spermatogenesis but testosterone is necessary for completing the process.

Hormonal changes : In bull calf, shortly after 2 months of age, there is pulsative discharge of LH. The concentrations of LH attain peak and decline upto about 6 months of age. From about 7 months to puberty the LH concentration increases linearly. Before 6 months of age, LH surges do not increase testosterone secretion from the testes indicating that Leydig's cells are not initially sensitive to LH. Later, the Leydig's cells become more and more sensitive to LH towards reaching the pubertal age. FSH levels are relatively constant and are free of episodic peaks. The FSH level does not change appreciably with age in males.

Spermatogenesis : Parallel to the endocrine changes leading to puberty in males, there are changes in the seminiferous tubules also. The sex cords are solid from birth to about 2 months of age and are composed of gonocytes and undifferentiated supporting cells. The spermatogonia first appear by about second month and are found nearly in all the tubules by about 5th month. The lumen formation in the seminiferous tubules starts by about 5.5 months and is completed by about 7.5 to 9.5 months. Sertoli cells are first observed by about 6.5 months. The primary spermatocytes first appear by about 5 months and the secondary spermatocytes first appear in between 5 and 6.5 months. The primary spermatocytes exceed that of spermatogonia by about 7.5 months. The spermadids appear in the seminiferous tubules by 6-7 months of age. The spermatozoa are seen only late in the prepubertal period. By about 9.5 month the undifferentiated supporting cells are changed to Sertoli cells. Secretion from accessory sex glands appears by 5 to 6 months.

Anatomical changes : The separation of penis from sheath starts by about 1 month of age. The separation proceeds caudally and is completed by about 8 months of age. The growth of the genital organs in very rapid from birth to 6 to 10 months of age. The penile growth is most rapid from birth to 6-7 months of age. The penile length increases up to nearly 5 times at the onset of puberty. The increase in penile length continues until sexual maturity. The sigmoid flexure begins to develop at about 3 months of age and becomes more and more prominent, thereafter.

Testicular development : The testicular growth is not appreciable upto 6 months of age. Thereafter, from 6 months to about 2 years of age the testicular development is very fast particularly during 10 to 20 months of age. By about 2-3 years of age, the testicles are developed to about 90% the mature size. Generally if the bull does not attain desired testicular growth by 2 years of age the chances for development at later stage are very remote.

FACTORS AFFECTING AGE AT PUBERTY AND SEXUAL MATURITY

The following factors may affect the age at puberty and sexual maturity in males :

1. Genetic factors
2. Nutritional factors
3. Hormonal factors
4. Social and climatic factors and
5. Body weight

Genetic factors : The pubertal age in males is the result of interaction between genetic and environmental factors. The variations in between species, breeds, strains and individuals clearly indicate that genetic factors influence age at puberty and sexual maturity. The zebu bulls reach puberty and sexual maturity about one year later than exotic breeds. Crossbred bulls attain puberty and sexual maturity earlier than the straightbred (inbred) bulls.

Nutritional factors : The nutrition of the animal plays a very vital role in affecting the age at puberty and sexual maturity in males. The nutrition of the animal should be maintained at optimum level starting from the birth. The deficiencies of TDN, protein, calcium, phosphorus, copper, cobalt, iron and iodine, etc. may prevent secretion of gonadotropins by the anterior pituitary gland. Proper growth of the animal is also important. The age at puberty and sexual maturity depends more on body weight (which is influenced by the level of nutrition) than to the age of the male. When the nutrition is good, the growth rate is faster and the animal attains puberty and sexual maturity at an early age. On the other hand, when the feeding level is low, the growth rate is slow and the males attain puberty and sexual maturity late. Males fed on too rich diet develop obesity and show delayed puberty and sexual maturity. The exact mechanism, as to how over feeding delays puberty and sexual maturity is not clearly understood. However, there may be following possibilities.

1. It may be possible that excessive fat around genital organs may interfere in the secretion of reproductive hormones or may absorb them from the blood stream. Thus, desirable amount of reproductive hormones may not be available for proper action.

2. Accumulation of fat around testes may form an insulating cover and thus may affect thermoregulation of the testes.

3. It is also possible that the obese bulls are lazy and sluggish and due to their physical inability, they may not show sexual interest.

Deficiencies of Vit-A may lead to irreversible degeneration of the seminiferous tubules. Deficiencies of Vit.-A, phosphorus and calcium may cause delay in the occurrence of puberty due to slow body growth rate.

Hormonal factors : The pituitary gonadotropins are present even in early post-natal life, but not in adequate quantity. In response to the secretion of gonadotropins from the anterior pituitary gland, testosterone levels rise from very low levels to adult levels. There is negative feed back mechanism in between testosterone. and gonadotropins. An optimal balance in the level of testosterone and gonadotropins is necessary for optimal functioning and hormonal imbalance may affect age at puberty and sexual maturity in males.

Social and climatic factors : Social and climatic factors also affect the age at puberty and sexual maturity in male animals. In rams, reduction in day light hours is followed by a decrease in prolactin and increase in gonadotropins and then by rise in testosterone level. Presence of the females of the same species generally hastens puberty in males. Extreme weather conditions like extreme cold and heat would depress sexual activity.

Body weight : The body weight of the animal is influenced by the level of the nutrition. As such the body weight of the animals is a good criterion for recommending the male for service. The average body weight, when the bulls be recommended for service should be nearly 240 kg and this weight must be gained by about 18 months of gage. In buffalo bulls the weight recommmende. to allow first service is around 280 kg.

LIBIDO

Libido means innate (inborn) sexual desire. Libido may be defined as willingness and eagerness to mount and attempt complete service. The reaction time is generally observed quite extensively to assess the sexual desire in AI bulls. Reaction time is measured as the time taken to collect the semen using artificial vagina by employing a non-estrous cow as mount animal in the crate for stimulus. Bulls reluctant to ejaculate within 15 minutes should be considered as problem cases. Generally good bulls donate semen within about 3 minutes. Nearly 25% of the bulls may have unacceptably long reaction time and hence it is important that the bulls be assessed for libido (reaction time) also. However, sex drive and mating ability has no relation with fertility in bulls. The sex drive is mainly hereditary in mature but may be modified by other factors. Males with strong sex drive do not easily change their mating behaviour and require greater insults from other physical and environmental factors to change their sexual instincts and behaviour. The various factors that influence the sex drive in bulls are :

1. Hereditary
2. Nutrition
3. Systemic diseases
4. Age
5. Management practices
6. Psychogenic factors
7. Climatic factors
8. Endocrine factors
9. Injuries of joints, muscles, nerves and tendon
10. Diseases of the penis and prepuce

Hereditary : Hereditary influence is most important in affecting the male's libido. Bulls with good libido produce more offsprings with good libido and bulls with poor libido produce more offsprings with poor libido. Similarities in sex drive are seen within twin pairs and differences in sex drive are seen in between twin pairs. The intensity of sex drive varies from breed to breed. Bulls of Indian breeds are poor in donating semen in artificial vagina. Bulls of Indian draught breeds (e.g. Hallikar and Amritmahal) have stronger sex drive compared to Indian milch breeds (e.g. Sahiwal and Sindhi). Males with stronger sex drive would require drastic and prolonged managemental and physical insults to change their sexual behaviour.

Nutrition : Males should be given properly balanced diet in adequate amount to maintain good body condition. Deficiencies of TDN, protein, phosphorus, calcium, copper, cobalt, iron, etc. would definitely influence the sex drive in males. Deficiencies, if are extremely enough, may lead to complete loss of libido. On the other hand overfed animals become obese, lazy and sluggish and are more prone to the problems of legs and joints. Feeding of excessive roughage leads to enlargement of rumen and abdomen and thus interfering with normal and easy copulation. Thus over feeding helps in the development of poor sex libido.

Systemic disease : Any disease causing depression, anorexia, fever, loss of weight and pain etc. would affect the sexual desire of the bull e.g.. Pneumonia, Enteritis, T.B., severe mange, severe parasitism, metastatic tumors, traumatic gastritis and severe peritonitis, etc. The extent of loss of sexual desire would depend upon the severity of the disease. All A.I. bulls should be watched carefully daily for the evidence of diseased conditions. The diagnosis and treatment of the disease should be done as quickly as possible to prevent loss of reproductive ability.

Age : Young and inexperienced bulls may not take interest in sexual activity. Older bulls may also show varying degree of lack of sexual desire. In young bulls reduced or lack of sexual desire is mostly due to deficiencies of nutrition. Low or subnormal feeding leads to delay in puberty and low sex drive. In older bulls a decrease in sex drive may be due to (1) decline in the level of testosterone, (2) senility, (3) loss of condition, (4) excessive use of male, and (5) arthritis etc.

Management : The sex drive also depends upon the way and the environment in which the bulls are trained, handled and managed. The bulls should always be handled carefully and with patience. Bulls become apprehensive about change of barn, change of attendants and the change of semen collection site. The timidness persists till the bulls adjust themselves to the new environment. Younger bulls isolated from other animals are easily frightened by the presence of other males and females and their activities. The timid young bulls which, are not experienced are generally slow to mount and copulate. Acquaintance of dog with bitch is necessary for copulation.

Psychogenic factors : The AI bulls should be reared in tension free environment. Inexperienced bulls kept in isolation are generally timid. The sex drive of the bull may decline with repeated frustration, harsh handling, abusive handling, punishment, abusive language, improper restraints, uncomfortable place, improper footing, painful experience in the past, low ceiling, inadequate space, lesions of the spinal column, too hot or too cold of artificial vagina, strange attendants, sudden noise, change of mount animal and with its too frequent use for semen collection. Presence of other bulls near the semen collection site stimulates sex drive.

Climatic factors : The climate has little or no effect on sex drive of native bulls and rams. During summer there is marked depression of sexual interests in buffalo bulls, exotic bulls and exotic rams.

Endocrine factors (Hypothyroidism, Hypogonadism or Pituitary deficiencies) : Though the deficiencies of thyroid, gonadal and pituitary hormones have not been proved clinically to be a cause for reduced sex drive, it is believed that poor libido may be due to deficiency of circulating androgens. It is possible that moderate deficiencies may cause reduction in sexual drive without other clinical symptoms.

Injuries of joints, muscles, nerves and tendon : Lesions affecting joints, muscles, nerves and tendons particularly affecting the rear quarter may affect sex drive.

Diseases of the penis and prepuce : The diseases of the penis and prepuce may be painful and hence may affect sex drive.

Chapter 4

Endocrine Control of Reproduction in Male Domestic Animals

The hormones control the reproduction even at the embryonic stage. In the developing embryo initially the gonads remain indifferent. Differentiation of the gonad into testis in male occur earlier compared to differentiation of gonad into ovary in female. Formation of tunica albuginea is the first histological evidence that the developing gonad would change into testis. The primitive testis apparently secretes androgen/androgen like substance which is responsible for (1) the development of the mesonephric tubules and ducts into permanent genital duct system of the male, (2) the formation of male's external genitalia and (3) the degeneration of the paramesonephric duct system.

Testicular descent : In females the ovaries remain in the abdominal cavity but in the males the testes descend into scrotum. The testicular descent is completed by birth or soon after and is also hormonally controlled by androgens from testes or adrenals. Thus the testes govern their own descent.

Before puberty : Prior to the onset of puberty releasing hormones are produced by the hypothalamus that cause the anterior pituitary gland to release gonadotropins from the basophilic cells (FSH, LH, TSH & ACTH are produced by basophilic and STH and LTH are produced by acidophils). The gonadotropic hormones (FSH and LH) are the same in males and females.

In females the relationship of the pituitary gonadotropins (FSH and LH) with ovary is cyclical but in males the relationship of pituitary gonadotropins with testis is not cyclical. The LH level fluctuates after birth and LH surges (Surge means an uprush) are noted but the LH surges do not increase testosterone secretion until the bulls are 6-7 months old indicating that Leydig cells are not sensitive to LH prior to this age. In males FSH does not appear to change appreciably with age.

GnRH and Gonadotropins : Gonadotropin releasing hormone (GnRH) is a decapeptide (pGlu-His-Trp-Ser-Tyr-Gly-Leu-Arg-Pro-Gly-NH$_2$) and stimulates the secretion of both FSH and LH. Both FSH and LH (also TSH) are glycoproteins and are made up of polypeptide chains or subunits (α subunit and β subunit—Fig. 4.1). There is non-covalent bonding in between the two

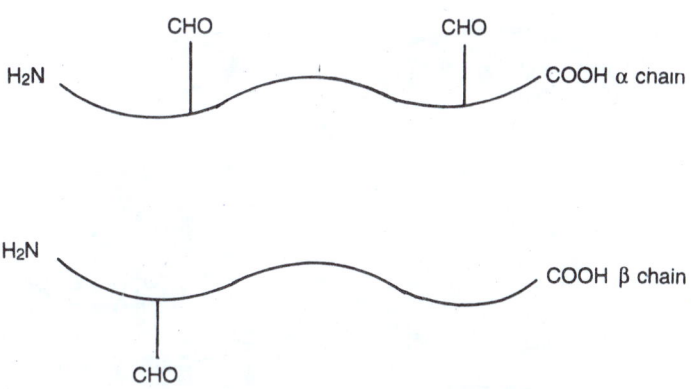

Fig. 4.1. α and β subunits of glycoprotein hormones.

- **Thyrotropin releasing hormone** is a tripeptide (pGlu-His-Pro-NH$_2$).
- **Corticotropin releasing hormone** is a 41 amino acid polypeptide.
- **Growth hormone releasing hormone** is a 44 amino acid polypeptide
- **Somatostatin** (inhibiting STH secretion) is a tetradecapeptide (Ala-Gly-Cys-Lys-Asn-Phe-Phe-Trp-Lys-Thr-Phe-Thr-Ser-Cys)

---

subunits. α subunit of oLH (Ovine LH) consists of 96 amino acids with 5 disulfide bonds and two carbohydrate chains. β subunit of oLH consists of 119 amino acids with 6 disulfide bonds and one carbohydrate chain. The α subunit is quite similar in between glycoprotein hormones and also in between species and is biologically inactive. The β subunit of the glycoprotein hormones is hormone and species specific and is biologically active. When the α and β subunit are separated, only the β subunit exhibits some very weak biological activity. Both the α and the β subunits in combined form are essential for full biological activity.

LH is required for spermatogenesis because it is required for the production of testosterone hormone. However, testosterone alone is not adequate for completion of spermatogenesis and a block on spermatogenesis occurs at meiosis : FSH is required for initial spermatogenesis. FSH is also important for the completion of meiosis and for final morphological differentiation of spermatid to spermatozoa through it influence on the activity of Sertoli cells. FSH also plays role in the release of spermatid from the syncytium of spermatids surrounding the Sertoli cells. There is some evidence that a third gonadotropin (prolactin) also plays an important role in the process of spermatogenesis. Prolactin facilitates the interaction of LH with its receptors located on Leydig cells (Fig. 4.2).

The Leydig cells and Sertoli cells : The Leydig cells are located outside the seminiferous tubules in the interstitium (Leydig cells are also called as interstitial cells). The Sertoli cells are large, have prominent nucleoli and are basely situated within the seminiferous tubule. Sertoli cells have long processes that surround spermatocytes and spermatids. The Sertoli cells provide nutrition and regulate the spermatogenesis. LH acts upon the Leydig cells (interstitial cells) of the testes, which in turn secrete testosterone. FSH acts upon Sertoli cells. Membrane receptors for FSH are present in the Sertoli cells. The cytoplasmic and nuclear receptors for androgens are also present in the Sertoli cells. The Sertoli cells are capable for following functions :

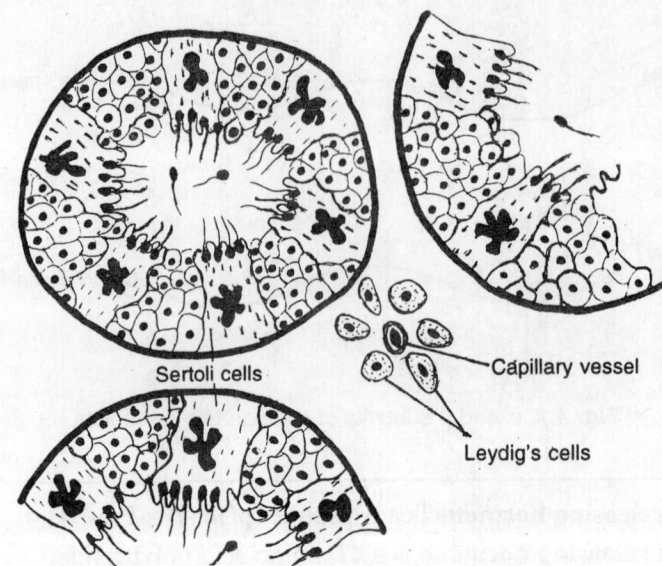

Fig. 4.2. Schematic section through seminiferous tubules to show Leydig's cells and Sertoli cells.

1. Sertoli cells may convert testosterone into estrogen. This situation is similar to females where testosterone produced by cells out side basement membrane (Theca layer) is converted into estrogen by the cells inside the basement membrane (Granulosa cells). Estrogens can move into both adluminal and basal compartments of the testis. From the basal compartment of the testis, estrogen may reach blood circulation where large quantity of estrogen may be detected, particularly in stallions. The specific role of estrogen on spermatogenesis is not clear.

2. The Sertoli cells are capable of converting testosterone into dihydrotestosterone, which has greater potency.

3. Sertoli cells can synthesize a specific androgen binding protein (ABP). Androgen binding with androgen binding proteins (ABP) helps in maintaining the concentration of androgens (testosterone and dihydrotestosterone) in the seminiferous tubules both for spermatogenesis and Sertoli cells function. Androgen binding protein may also be responsible for transporting testicular androgens into the epididymis.

4. Sertoli cells also produce inhibin (Protein hormone, having α and β subunits and β subunit is important for its biological activity) that suppresses the production of FSH from the anterior pituitary gland.

The steroid hormones : The gonadal steroids are lipid hormones having a common *cyclopentanoperhydrophenanthrene* nucleus (perhydro means that hydrogen has been added to the double bond) which contains 3 six membered phenanthrene rings and 1 five membered cyclopentane ring (Fig. 4.3). The basic cyclopentanoperhydrophenanthrene nucleus contains 17 carbon atoms. The C-10 and C-13 are generally attached to the methyl groups. Wide varieties of side chains are attached at C-17.

Steroidogenesis : Cholesterol is probably the basic substance for the synthesis of steroid hormones. Cholesterol is transported to mitochondria where cleavage in the side chain between C-20 and C-22 occurs and pregnanolone is formed. Pregnanolone is converted in to progesterone

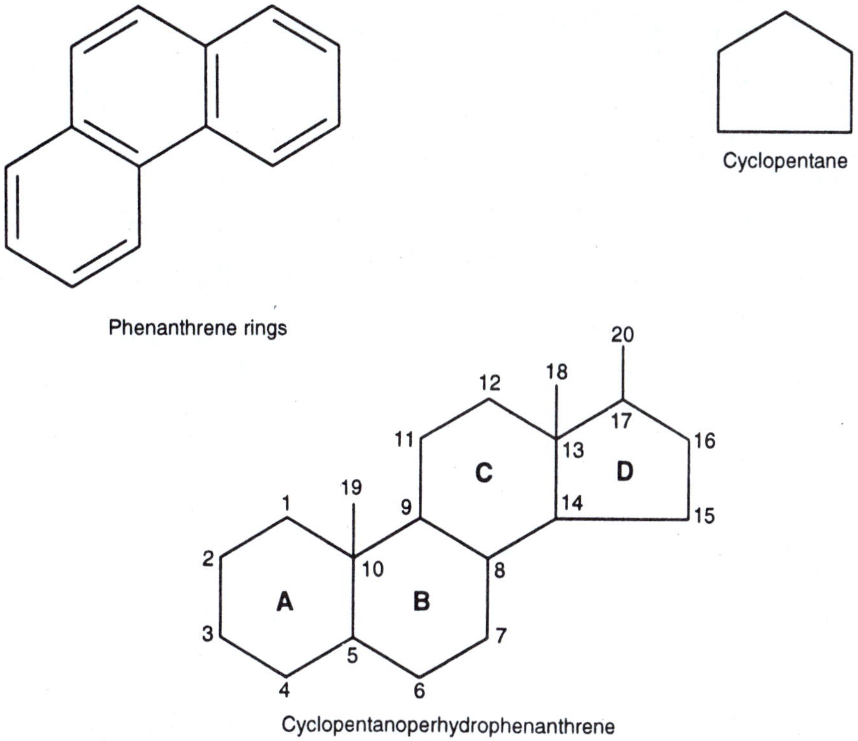

Cyclopentane

Phenanthrene rings

Cyclopentanoperhydrophenanthrene

- A, B and C are six-membered phenanthrene rings
- D is five-membered Cyclopentane ring
- C-18 and C-19 are methyl groups at C-13 and C-10 respectively
- C-20 and C-21 project as side chain from C-17
- Perhydro means that hydrogen has been added to the double bond

Fig. 4.3. Cyclopentanoperhydrophenanthrene skeleton of steroid hormones.

in the endoplasmic reticulum. Androgens from progesterone are formed in the cytoplasm. Multiple enzymes are required for the biosynthesis of steroid hormones and the enzymes are located at various subcellular levels. Estrogens are produced from androgens by eliminating C-19 methyl group. The biosynthesis of steroid hormones from cholesterol is depicted in Fig. 4.4. The structures of some synthetic hormones are shown in Fig. 4.5.

PHYSIOLOGICAL ACTIONS OF ANDROGENS

1. Sexual differentiation of male duct system and external male genitalia
2. Testicular descent.
3. Androgens is essential for libido.
4. Androgens are required for normal spermatogenesis.
5. Maintenance of secretory and absorptive activity of efferent ducts, epididymis and vas deferens including ampullae.
6. Androgens are required for maintaining structural and secretory activity of the accessory sex glands including seminal vesicles, prostate and bulbourethral glands.

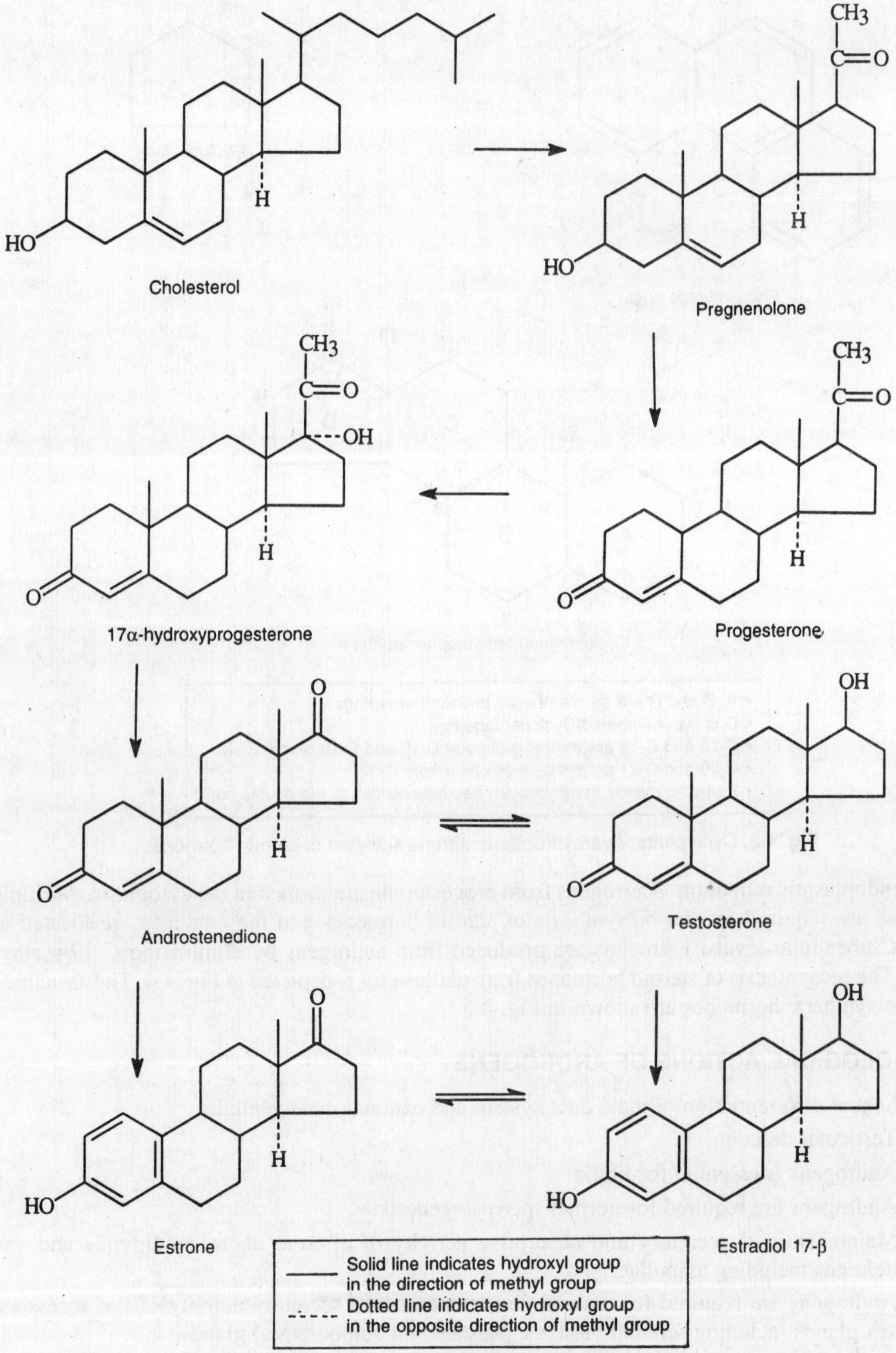

Fig. 4.4. Biosynthesis of steroid hormones from cholesterol.

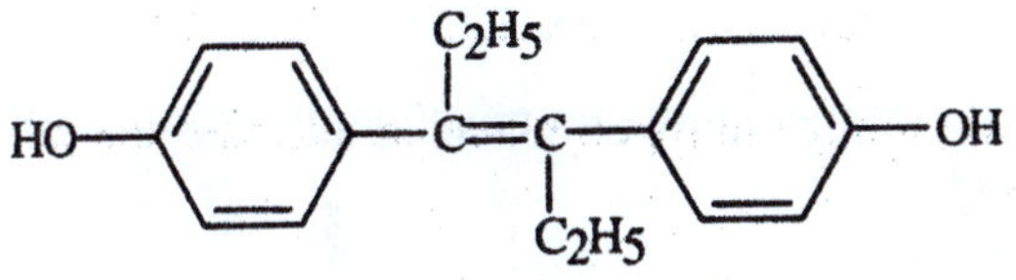

Diethylstilbestrol

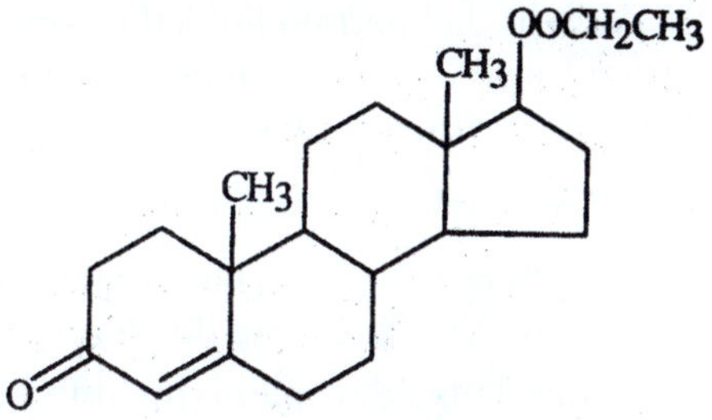

Testosterone propionate

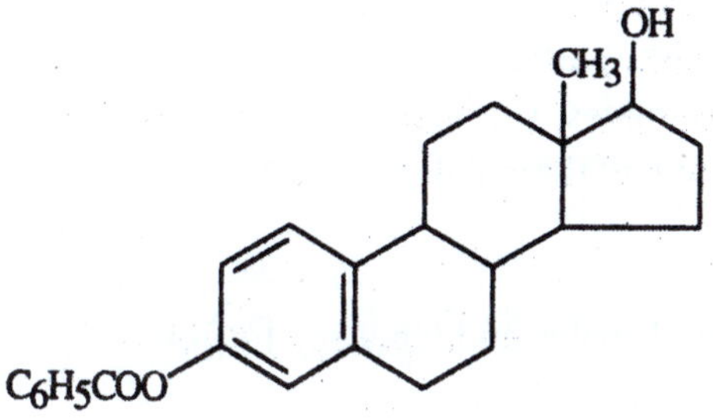

Estradiol benzoate

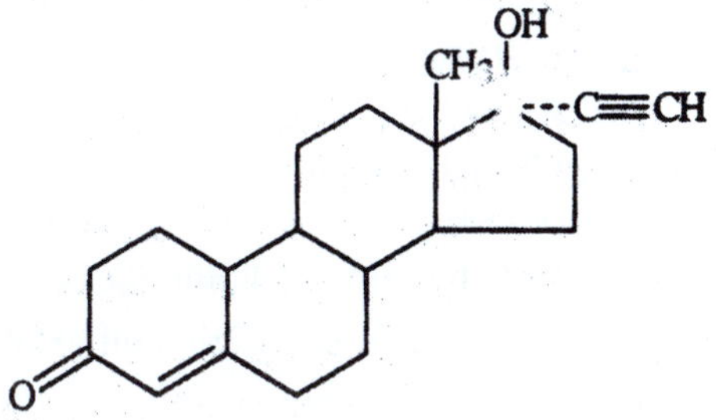

Norgestomet

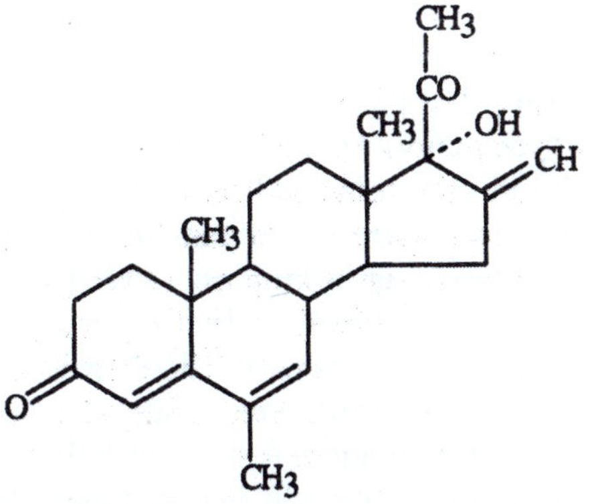

Melengestrol acetate

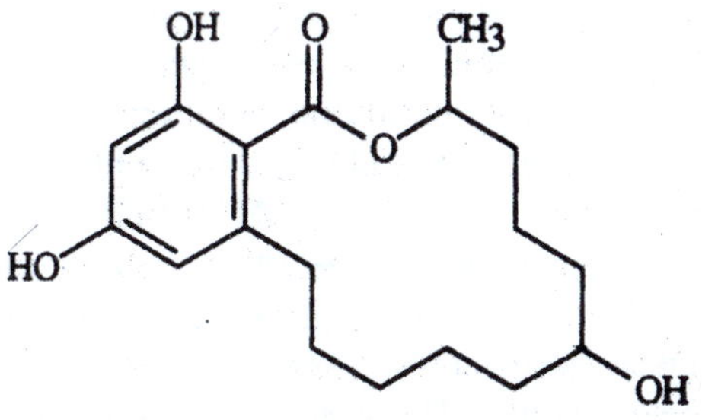

Zeranol

Fig. 4.5. Some synthetic hormones.

In bulls and buffalo bulls the seminal fructose is mainly derived from vesicular glands. The initial fructose content in the semen is indicative of the activity of Leyding cells and sex drive. The rate of fructolysis helps to determine semen quality.

7. Androgens have protein anabolic effects and promote nitrogen retention, increase the number of muscle fibres and thickness in the males.
8. It prolongs the epididymal life of the sperms.
9. Androgens stimulate growth of the penis and scrotum.
10. Androgens are responsible for keratinisation of preputial epithelium.
11. Androgens are responsible for separation of glans penis from the prepuce.
12. Urinary patterns in male dogs (raising of one hind limb) is due to testosterone.
13. Marking of a territory by male dogs is by substances known as pheromones that are produced by kidney under the influence of testosterone.
14. Secondary sexual characteristics specific to males are due to androgens e.g..
    (a) Distribution of body hairs (e.g. beard) and horn growth.
    (b) Bigger appearance of males compared to females. (in females estrogen acts upon epiphyseal cartilage of long bones) together with increase in muscle mass through retention of nitrogen (protein anabolic effect)
    (c) Development of hump and shoulder.
    (d) Aggressive, energetic and excitable nature of males and tendency to fight.
    (e) Tough skin (not so soft as in females).
    (f) Deep pitched voice in males compared to females.

Overstimulation of interstitial cells by pituitary gonadotropins may lead to excessive testosterone production. In dog this may lead to hypertrophy and hyperplasia of prostate gland. This may cause compression of rectum, constipation, tenesmus (painful and ineffectual straining to relieve the bowels) and perineal hernia.

OTHER HORMONES

The contractile mechanisms involved in the sperm transport are partly controlled by oxytocin. Oxytocin injected in males prior to ejaculation results in hyperspermia (increased ejaculate volume) and polyzoospermia (increased sperm concentration). There are some indications that prostaglandins influence epididymal contractions (oxytocic affect) and hence sperm transport. There are some indication, that PG $F_2 \alpha$ is implicated in the release of gonadotropins. Other pituitary hormones (e.g.. TSH, STH, ACTH and Vasopressin), thyroid hormones, adrenal corticoids etc. have only moderate and secondary role on the reproduction in male animals. The thyroid gland has some indirect, if not direct role in male reproduction. Thyroidectomized bulls lose sexual interest in estrous cows. Seasonal changes in the thyroid secretion and the testes of buffalo bulls have been noted. There are indications that there is a definite threshold below which thyroid secretions should not drop if the reproduction is to be retained normal in males. Thyroproteins prevent drop in spermatozoa production in hot weather and thiouracil (inhibitor of thyroid secretion) causes drop in sperm production.

Chapter 5

Sexual Behaviour in Male Animals

The animals are mostly social ones and prefer living in herds. In each species there are certain rules for group survival, cohesion, defense and also for propagation. The basic patterns of male sexual behaviour appear to be innate in nature. Calves of both sexes are very often seen exhibiting sexual display during play and mounting is seen most commonly. Bulls reared in complete isolation show normal mating behaviour when exposed to estrous cows. In females the sexual receptivity is restricted to few hours or days near the estrous phase of the estrous cycle, while in males the sexual receptivity is grossly permanent. The physiological signals for arousal of sexual motivations originate from gonadal steroid balance. However, the secretion of gonadal steroids is not permanent. In males the androgen secretion is in the form of several peaks within 24 hours reflecting the pulsative release of pituitary gonadotropins. However, the total amount of androgen in males is almost constant practically for day to day. In females the secretions of estrogens are restricted only during few days (follicular phase) of the estrous cycle.

The various components of copulatory patterns in male domestic animals are :

1. Sexual arousal
2. Courtship (sexual display)
3. Erection.
4. Penile protrusion.
5. Mounting.
6. Intromission.
7. Ejaculation.
8. Dismounting and
9. Refractoriness.

Each response becomes a stimulus for next component of the copulatory pattern. The events of courtship and copulation are shorter in cattle, sheep and goat (one second or so) and are longer in swine (about 5 minutes or even more) and horse (about 40 seconds). The sexual responses in cattle, sheep and goats are shown in Figs. 5.1, 5.2 and 5.3.

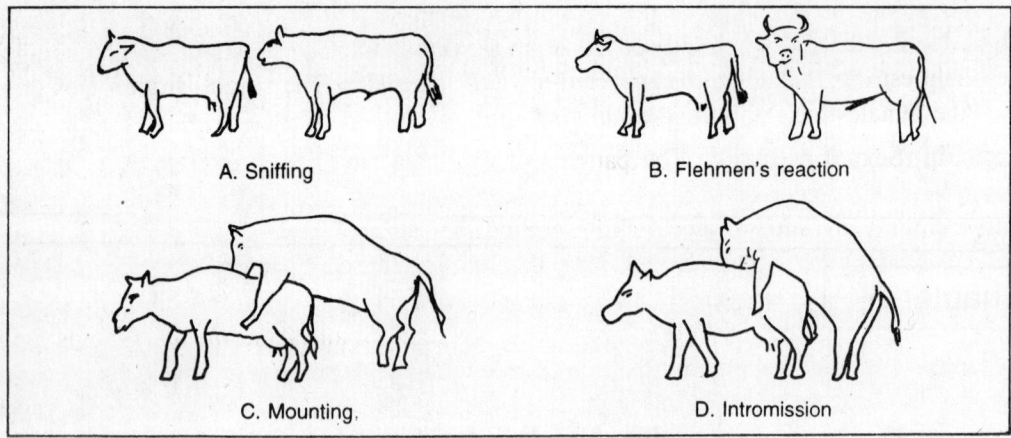

Fig. 5.1. Sexual responses in cattle.

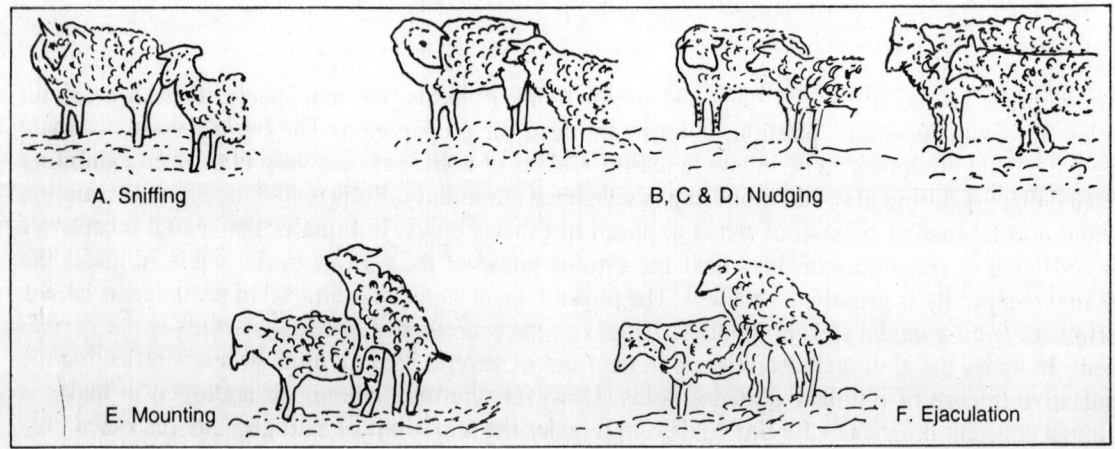

Fig. 5.2. Sexual responses in sheep.

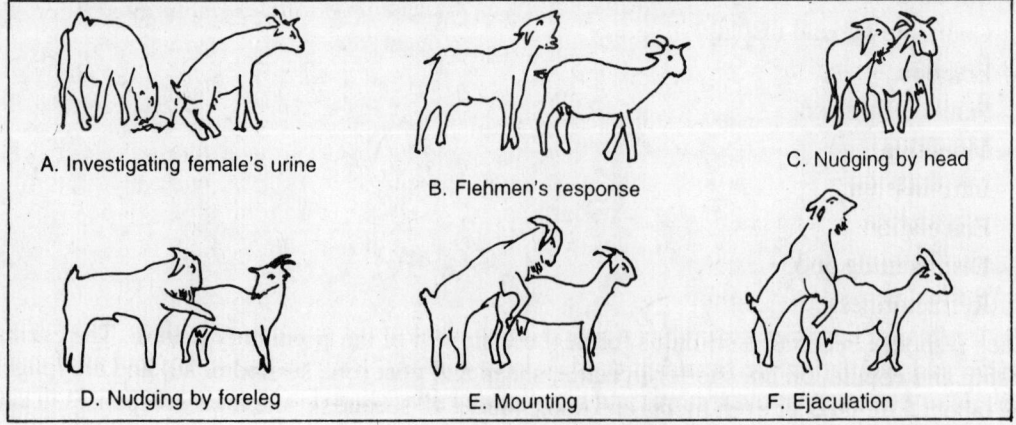

Fig. 5.3. Sexual responses in goat.

Sexual arousal : The finding of the sexual partner is the first step for sexual arousal and in that all the senses like sight, hearing and olfaction are important. The senses of sight, hearing and olfaction help estrous females to be attracted towards the males. The stimuli from males greatly influence the females for exhibiting sexual responses.

Courtship (Sexual display) : The patterns of courtship are simple in domestic animals but species specific differences do occur. Once attracted to a female partner, the bull tests her receptivity most oftenly by sniffing and licking around the perineal region. These actions indicate chemical communication in between the male and female partners. Sniffing to female's genitalia and urine is very commonly seen in cattle, sheep and goat. Sniffing to females head is commonly seen in swine and horses. Following sniffing to female's genitalia and urine, the male stands rigidly, makes the head in horizontal position with neck extended and the upper lips are curled upward to perform the **"Flehmen's reaction"**. Flehmen's reaction is seen in all species except in swine. Characteristic odour does not appear to play a role during courtship. However, species specific patterns of urination during court ship are noticed in some species. Stallion marks with urine the place where an estrous mare has urinated. There is rhythmic emission of urine during sexual activity. In goats, frequent miction on forelegs is seen during sexual activity. Urination during sexual excitement has not been observed in cattle and sheep.

Vocalization species specific vocalization patterns are also observed in males during courtship. Courting bleats are noticed in male sheep and goat during sexual display. Courting grunts are observed in swine. Neighing is observed in horses during sexual excitement. In bulls no vocalization patterns are observed during sexual display.

Nudging (Nudge = to push gently specially to draw attention) and licking of the females external genitalia and perineal region are noticed in cattle, sheep and goat. Nudging of the female through forelegs is commonly seen in sheep and goat. Nudging through nosing the flank area of the female is observed in swine. The stallion bites over the mare's back and neck and also licks the mare's body.

Erection and penile protrusion : The vascular penis in the stallion and dog erects slowly and there is foreplay before copulation. The penis of bull, ram and boar is fibroelastic and the vascular tissue is much less and there is varying amount of foreplay in these species. The erection process is predominantly under the control of parasympathetic system. Reflex stimulations from testicles, urethra, prostate or penis and specially the glans penis cause erection. The acts of erection and ejaculation are reflex with centers being located in the lumber region of the spinal cord and also involve cerebral cortex of the brain.

The penis of the sexually active male may erects partially and there may be to and fro penile movements before mounting. During this process dribblings of accessory fluid derived from the Cowper's gland may also be seen, especially in bulls. The male rests his chin on female's body and the receptive female respond by standing quietly in order to allow mounting by the male.

Mounting : The sexually active male mounts the female. Some initial mounts may be unsuccessful with excretion of dribblings. During this process the movements of bull's hind limbs and contractions of his abdominal muscles particularly the rectus abdominis muscle align the glans penis both horizontally and vertically to seek vulva for penetration. The male mounts, grasps the female by fixing fore legs around female's body. During this process rhythmic pelvic thrusts may be performed (Fig. 5.4).

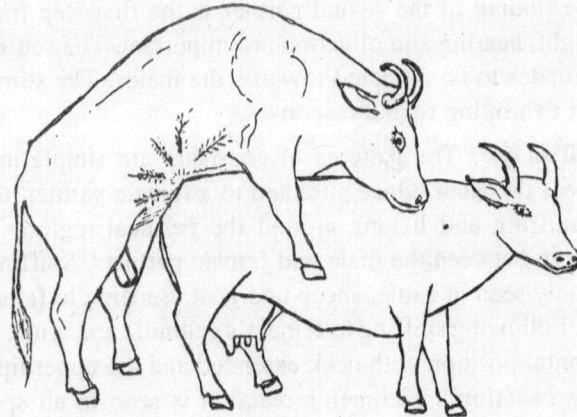

Fig. 5.4. Mounting and intromission by bull. The male grasps the female's body by fixing forelegs around female's body and there is contraction of abdominal muscles, particularly the rectus abdominis muscle.

> The mounting has been widely exploited in semen collection from bulls. Practically the greatest stimulus for bull to ejaculate is the female's rear quarter or something similar to it. Even male dummies are satisfactorily utilized for semen collection. However, the mounting object should be at appropriate height, should have adequate strength and should have immobility.

Intromission : In farm animals one Intromission takes places per copulation. At mounting, the male's pelvic region is brought in close apposition to the female's external genitalia. The movements of the male help the glans penis to seek vulva. The vulvar heat and moisture are detected by the superficial nerve endings of the glans penis and this sensation is the leading factor for proper Intromission. Stallion oscillates the pelvis several times which causes engorgement of penis with blood and thus making it rigid for intromission. Full intromission of the penis occurs after ejaculatory thrust. The duration of the intromission varies greatly in between different species. The intromission is instant in bull, ram and goat. Boars on average take 5 minutes per mating, however, they may maintain intromission up to 20 minutes. Horses maintain intromission on an average for 40 seconds.

Ejaculation : The ejaculation after intromission is dependent upon the nerve impulses from the dorsum of the free portion of the penis. Generalized muscular contractions. especially of abdominal muscles take place at ejaculation. The process of ejaculation start from epididymis, travel along ductus deferens and at the same time accessory sex glands contract and their contents are forced into urethra. Oxytocin is released and causes transport of semen in the epididymis and ductus deferens. Rhythmic contractions of the urethral, ischiocavernosus and bulbocavernosus muscles cause release of semen from urethra. At ejaculation there is maximum lengthening of the penis so that the semen is ejaculated near os cervix in case of cattle, sheep and goat; in the cervix and uterus in boar and in the uterus in horse. At ejaculation the bull leaps and the thrust is very strong. Bulls often coil the penis during ejaculation. At ejaculation in sheep and goat, the male's head is suddenly moved backward. The bull at ejaculation presses its head on female's back. The boar remains motionless during ejaculation, however, scrotal contractions are observed. During such period of immobility some thrusts at irregular intervals are seen in boar. In horses the male bites the female's neck.

Dismounting : After the ejaculation has taken place, the male dismounts and soon the penis is withdrawn into the prepuce. Postcoital display are rare in domestic animals. Postcoital reactions are generally not seen in cattle, swine and horse. The male goat licks the penis after ejaculation. The male sheep stretches its head and neck after ejaculation.

Refractoriness : Most of the males would not show sexual interest in females immediately following copulation and this is known as refractoriness. The period of refractoriness varies greatly in between individual males. Repeated and successive copulations greatly increase the period of refractoriness. The period of refractoriness is modified by environmental stimuli e.g.. male to female ratio, cyclicity of the female, length of the breeding season and social interactions among animals. The presentation of new stimuli can revitalize sexual interest in males. Generally, the approach of the male towards the female is selective in nature. The goat, boar and stallion reach exhaustion after smaller number of ejaculations than ram and bull. The pasture-mated bulls may perform 30-35 services per day provided stimulus is adequate. After long period of sexual rest, a ram may perform up to 50 services on first day but this frequency would greatly reduce on subsequent days.

Chapter 6

Infertility in Male Animals

Infertility or lower fertility in males, particularly in bulls had long been considered to be a rare occurrence, but now infertility in males in being considered to be a common and severe problem, Still there is paucity of information concerning the male's infertility.

FORMS OF INFERTILITY IN THE MALE

The forms of infertility in the males may be divided into the following 3 main categories, though there may be some overlapping.

1. Reduced or complete lack of sexual desire and ability to copulate (Impotentia coeundi)
2. Inability or reduced ability to fertilize (Impotentia generandi)
3. Miscellaneous diseases affecting the reproductive organs.

The above conditions are present in the males of all the species and the conditions may vary in degree from mild to severe forms. Libido (sex drive) is generally not related to fertility in males and the semen of bull with low sex drive may have excellent fertility. Examination of the male for infertility/sterility should be done very carefully for its proper treatment/disposal. For investigating the accurate cause of male's infertility, following examinations are essential.

1. Breeding and health records of the male and also of the herd.
2. Critical examination of the male including its mating behaviour.
3. Thorough examination of the semen by trained veterinarian/personnel.

IMPOTENTIA COEUNDI (REDUCED TO COMPLETE LACK OF SEXUAL DESIRE AND ABILITY TO COPULATE)

In females the reproductive behaviour in rather simple, compared to males. In females only the willingness to stand and to be mounted is required. In males, the reproductive behaviour is rather more complex and requires identification and seeking of the female together with complete act of copulation. Hence, in males complete physical capability is necessary so that each component of copulatory patterns (sexual arousal, sexual display, erection of penis, protrusion of penis, mounting, intromission and dismounting etc) are performed well. Hence, it is necessary that all senses of the male including visual, olfactory, auditory, and tactile etc. should be perfectly normal.

FACTORS AFFECTING THE SEX DRIVE

The different factors affecting the sex drive are (1) Hereditary, (2) Nutrition, (3) Systemic diseases, (4) Age, (5) Managemental practices, (6) Psychogenic factors, (7) Climatic factors, (8) Endocrine factors, (9) Joint, muscle, bone, nerve and tendon injuries, (10) Diseases of penis and prepuce (e.g. Balanoposthitis, phimosis, paraphimosis, diphallus, phallocampsis, adhesions of the penis and prepuce, ruptured or broken penis, tumors of the penis and prepuce) and (11) certain miscellaneous causes e.g. Hernias, premature erection, loss of sensory innervation of the glans penis, urinary caliculi and other causes (refer libido, Chapter 3).

PROGNOSIS

The prognosis of Impotentia coeundi (reduced to complete lack of sexual desire and ability to copulate) is generally guarded to poor. Low sex drive of genetic origin is impossible to be improved. However, low sex drive due to environmental factors and due to curable ailments is possible to overcome. The prognosis of the males with joint, muscle, tendon, bone or nerve injuries would depend upon the nature and severity of the condition and the value of the animal.

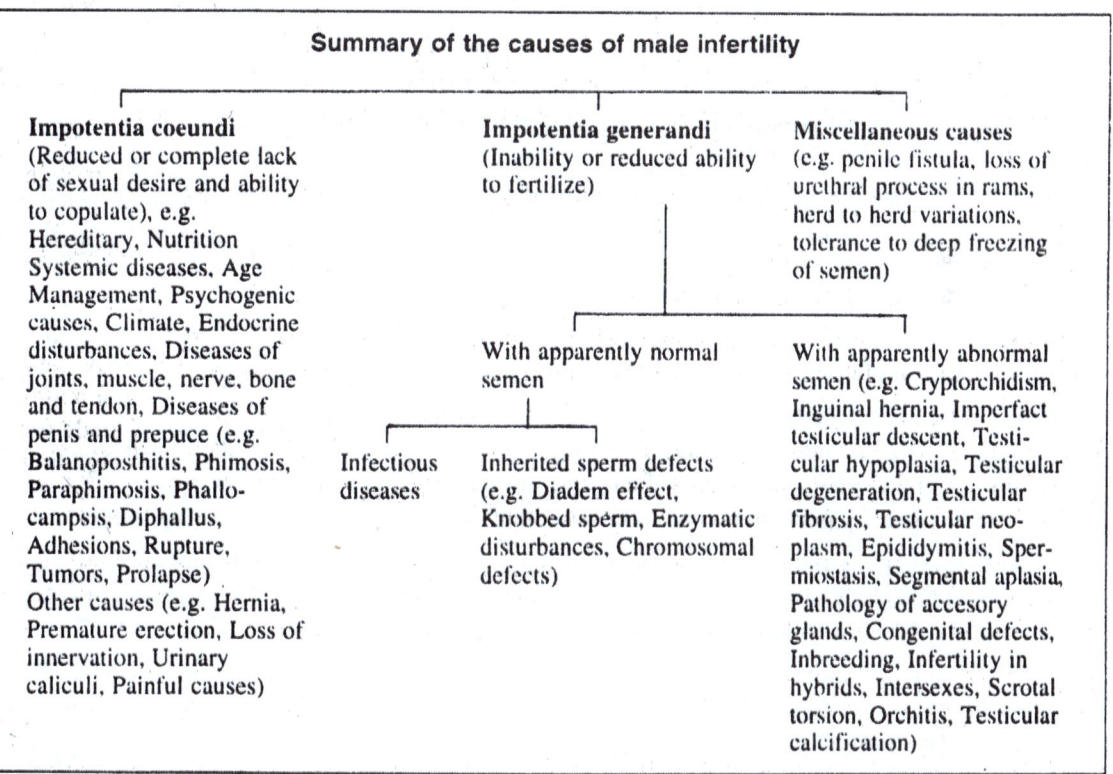

TREATMENT

Since the causes of impotentia coeundi are variable, there cannot be a single treatment for curing the condition. The treatment of this condition with drug and hormones is of questionable value and should not be resorted to, in general. It is imperative (urgently necessary) to carefully find out for certain the cause of the problem before starting the treatment. Before starting treatment it is necessary that following should be done.

1. Carefully collect and study the breeding history.

2. The physical examination of the bull should be conducted thoroughly.

3. Carefully examine the male during coitus for its serving ability. The serving ability of the male may be examined repeatedly, if required.

4. Special attention should be paid to examine nutrition, diseases, managemental practices, exercise, and psychic pressure on the male and the conditions that may be pain-striking to the males.

The animals, which are thin and emaciated and are suffering from deficiencies of TDN, Protein, vitamins and certain minerals (e.g. phosphorus and cobalt), may have reduced libido. Low energy levels retard puberty as well as libido in males. On the contrary over fed males become obese and lazy and very often suffer with problems of joints and foot. Excessive feeding of roughages leads to the enlargement of rumen and abdomen and interferes in easy copulation. Males should be provided with balanced nutritive diet and should be given sufficient exercise so that their body remains in a fairly good condition.

The diseases, if any, resulting in loss of body weight, anorexia, weakness, depression and loss of sexual desire, should be thoroughly investigated and treated accordingly. Parasitism should be examined and alleviated. Early diagnosis and prompt treatment of diseases are indicated to prevent loss of reproductive ability in males.

Sexual load on males should be examined. If the bulls are overused, the frequency of services may be reduced or the males may be given sexual rest. Young and inexperienced males may show reduced sexual interests. In older bulls sexual interests may be reduced due to loss of condition. The conditions should be handled accordingly.

Size as well as nature of the dummy should be examined. Size of dummy is important for mounting and ejaculation by the male. The dummy should be of docile nature.

Bull should always be handled with patience. Inexperienced and timid bulls are slow to mount and copulate. The surroundings should be conducive e.g. pleasant atmosphere, adequate room, good footing and friendly attendants. Fear and apprehension are hostile (unfriendly) for sexual expression. Change of place and change of attendants should be avoided as far as possible.

Males experiencing pain or punishment during sex may decline to donate semen. Only skilled operators should be allowed to collect semen using artificial vagina. Artificial vagina should neither be too hot nor too cold and should have adequate pressure.

Change of mount animal and longer "teasing" period may be helpful in slow breeders. Poor libido is thought to be due to deficiency in circulating androgens, but on many occasions, the concentration of circulating testosterone is found to have no relation with libido, making the treatment questionable with hormones. Oily preparations of testosterone may be used .

Bull and stallion	100-500 mg	Repeated at
Boar and ram	50-100 mg	weekly
Dog	10-50 mg	intervals

Prolonged therapy with testosterone should be avoided as it may lead to atrophy and degeneration of testes because of suppression of gonadotropic hormones.

One or more injections of chorionic gonadotropins may also be used.

Large animals	5000-10000 I.U. i/m or s/c
Dog and other small animals	100-500 I.U. i/m or s/c

Chorionic gonadotropins help production of testosterone by the interstitial cells.

Males that are obese and lazy possibly because of deficiency of thyroid hormones may be fed iodinated casein @ 2 gm/100 kg body weight. This may increase metabolic rate and may prevent loss of libido.

Diseases affecting joint, muscle, nerve, bone and tendon should be treated accordingly. Inflammation particularly affecting the rear quarter may cause impotentia coeundi. Other conditions e.g. foot rot, over grown claws and hooves, interdigital necrosis, traumatic lesions, spinal diseases may also cause pain and hence reduced libido. The treatment in such conditions would depend upon the nature and severity of the condition and the value of the animal. In most cases sexual rest, restriction of movements enforced by confinement in small paddock and providing proper footings are indicated. As supportive treatment, balanced feeding, application of counter irritants and massage may be indicated in some cases. Interdigital necrosis should be removed surgically. Trimming of hooves should be done to make them symmetrical. Infections or traumatic lesions should be appropriately handled. Tranquilizers may also be helpful in treatment of bulls but such bulls should be carefully looked upon so that they do not injure themselves upon rising. Glucocorticoids may also be of supportive value in alleviating signs of arthritis. In valuable bulls semen may be obtained by electro-ejaculation technique.

Balanitis (inflammation of the glans penis), posthitis (inflammation of the prepuce), balanoposthitis (inflammation of the penis and prepuce), phimosis (animal is unable to normally protrude the penis), paraphimosis (animal is unable to retract the penis into the prepuce), diphallus (double penis and normal copulation would be prevented because of forked configuration), phallocampsis (deviation of the penis either ventral or lateral or spiral or corkscrew type), a persistent frenulum (a band of tissue extending from near the ventral tip of the penis to the prepuce), adhesions of the penis and prepuce, ruptured or broken penis, tumors of the penis and prepuce, chronic prolapse of the prepuce, and also some miscellaneous factors are common causes of failure for successful copulation and result in marked loss of sexual desire. These conditions are discussed under separate headings.

Balanoposthitis

Often the inflammations of the penis and prepuce are involved together (balanoposthitis) because of the close anatomical relationship. The condition may be due to infectious or non-infectious causes. In balanoposthitis, the copulation is usually prevented due to stenosis of the prepucial orifice, adhesions between the penis and prepuce or due to pain. Wide variety of organisms including bacteria, moulds, protozoa and viruses are found in the prepucial cavity e.g. E. coli, Streptococci, Staphylococci, B. pyocyaneus, P. aeruginosa, C. pyogenes, Proteus, Actinomycetes necrophorus, Actinobaccilli, Micobacterium tuberculosis, Molds (Aspergillus, Mucor, Absidia), Mycoplasma and IBR-IPV virus. With trauma, lacerations, abrasions etc. of the glans penis and prepuce the above organisms may enter the deeper tissue resulting in inflammation with swelling, discharge and pain. Faulty methods of semen collection with artificial vagina may cause lacerations of the glans. Hairs may be drawn in the prepuce during homosexual behaviour in young bulls. Most of the times recovery is usually spontaneous.

Prognosis : The prognosis of the balanoposthitis depends upon severity of trauma or infection. The prognosis is good in mild cases and guarded in chronic cases with severe adhesions in between the penis and prepuce.

Treatment : The treatment in mild cases consists of douching the prepuce with antiseptics (1 :2000 acriflavin or potassium permanganate solution; 1 per cent hydrogen peroxide solution) or antibiotics. Irritant antiseptics should be avoided. Application of oily preparations of antiseptics and antibiotics together with gentle protrusion of the penis may aid in preventing possible adhesions. Systemic antibiotics should also be given in severe cases. Tranquilizers, anesthetics, pudental nerve block and adequate restraints may be desirable in applying the treatment. Sexual rest during treatment and for sometime thereafter is essential to avoid pain and to promote recovery.

Phimosis or stenosis of prepucial orifice

Phimosis or stenosis of the prepucial orifice leads to prevention of normal protrusion of the penis and thus the male is unable to perform coitus.

The causes of phimosis or stenosis of prepucial orifice may be (1) Congenital (especially in dog, cat and horses) and (2) acquired due to injuries, wounds and infections.

The prognosis is guarded and depends upon extent of trauma, necrosis and the promptness of handling the case.

The phimosis of congenital origin may be corrected by surgical operation. Other cases may be treated by conventional methods.

Paraphimosis

Paraphimosis is the inability of the penis to be retracted back into the prepuce after protrusion resulting into swelling, oedema and balanoposthitis. The causes of paraphimosis are :

1. Secondary to swelling and oedema of prepuce.
2. Paralysis of the penis due to spinal diseases, and
3. After resection (cutting away) retractor penis muscle in bulls.

The prognosis in paraphimosis is guarded and depends upon degree of trauma, degree of necrosis and the promptness of treatment.

The treatment consists of careful cleaning of the penis, removal of the necrotic tissue and liberal use of broad-spectrum antibiotic ointments. Cold packs may help reduce swelling. Sometimes, it may be imperative (urgently necessary) to surgically enlarge the prepucial opening in order to replace the penis, The penis should be wrapped with gauze and the penis with its gauge dressing should be replaced inside sheath as soon as possible. Liberal use of oily ointments or vaseline with daily withdrawal of penis would prevent adhesions. Support of prolapsed penis and sheath using tight suspensory bandage would help minimize the oedema. In severe cases amputation of the penis is recommended.

Diphallus

Diphallus (double penis) prevents normal copulation because of forked configuration.

Phallocampsis

Phallocampsis or deviation of the penis either ventral (rainbow deviation), lateral or corkscrew type or due to a congenitally persistent frenulum is a common cause for difficulty in copulation and loss of libido.

The deviation of the penis due to congenitally persistent frenulum may be easily corrected by cutting the connective tissue band causing deviation of the penis. Other types of penile deviation may be corrected surgically but not always satisfactorily.

Adhesions of the penis and prepuce

Adhesions in the region of the sigmoid flexure may be due to horn injuries in bull and ram and due to these adhesions normal penile protrusion in prevented. Surgical treatments of these adhesions often leads to more severe form of adhesions. Deeper adhesions in the region of the fornix produce more severe phimosis compared to the adhesions in the cranial portion of the prepuce. Vigorous thrust during semen collection with artificial vagina may produce injury or even tear the prepuce or injure the circumference of the penis. Subsequent infections may produce abscesses and may even produce adhesions. In such cases prompt treatment with antibiotics both locally in oily base and as well as by parenteral route is indicated along with complete sexual rest during treatment and for sometime thereafter as discussed under phimosis.

Ruptured or broken penis

A ruptured or fractured or broken penis is usually observed in younger bulls with strong sex drive. The injury usually occurs at the time of coitus when the cow suddenly goes down or suddenly falls under the weight of the bull or the erected penis is bended due to strike on abnormal site on cow at the movement of bull thrust. The site of rapture of the penis is generally behind the attachment of the retractor penis muscle. Rarely the condition may occur in stallion due to kicking by mare on erected penis. In dog the fracture of the penis may be caused by traumatic injuries.

The symptoms of the rupture of the penis are arching of back, short strides, stiffness, and pain and swelling cranial to scrotum. There may be oedema, which may later develop into hard mass. Because of the very high blood pressure in the erect corpus cavernosum penis, the haemorrhage on fracture of penis is profuse. Initially the swelling is soft and fluctuating but as the blood clots it becomes hard. There may be pain but heat is only slight. Such bulls usually become unfit for breeding.

Tumors of the penis and prepuce

Tumors in the penis and prepuce have been observed in bull, stallion and dog. These tumors may be single or multiple and are firm and cauliflower like growths. These tumors may lead to phimosis, paraphimosis, haemorrhage after service and also hesitancy or even refusal to serve.

In bull, the prognosis is comparatively good, particularly if the tumor is not multiple. After pudental block or tranquilizers and local anesthesia the penis is withdrawn from the sheath and the tumor is removed surgically. The mucus membrane of the penis and/or prepuce are sutured with fine cat gut. In stallion, generally the amputation of the penis is recommended. In dog, tumor may be removed surgically. In all cases after surgery prompt treatment with antibiotics locally in only base as well as by parenteral routes for several days are indicated. All such animals be given sexual rest during treatment and for some time thereafter.

Chronic prolapse of the prepuce

Chronic prolapse of the prepuce is probably an inherited condition associated with pendulous sheath and a large prepucial orifice. The condition is most commonly seen in bulls of Indian milch breeds like Sahiwal and Sindhi. In Indian draught breeds like Hallikar, Hariana and Malva, the sheath is usually tucked up and the prolapse of the prepuce is uncommon. It is less commonly seen in exotic breeds of cattle. In affected bulls, the pendulous sheath may be easily traumatized, lacerated, infected and may become frost-bitten, inflamed, oedematous, and fibrotic.

For treatment, the affected bull may be confined to a clean, hygienic and comfortable stall. The prolapsed organ should be thoroughly washed, cleaned and dried. Broad spectrum antibiotics in oily base are applied in the affected area. The prolapse is replaced and is held in position by purse-string suture through the prepucial orifice. Antibiotics may also be given by parenteral route as per need and repeated dressings may be required for 3-4 weeks. In more severe cases in which replacement is not possible amputation of the prepuce may be necessary.

Other causes of loss of libido and inability to copulate

Hernias

Hernias and even bulky abdomen may affect penetration of the penis into vagina. Both the umbilical and ventral hernias may be corrected surgically but since the umbilical hernia may be hereditary, such animal should be culled and should not be used for breeding purpose. Too much feeding of roughage causes extensive abdominal size and in such animals roughage feeding should be markedly reduced.

Premature erection

In certain bulls premature full erection causes corkscrewing and coiling of the free end of the penis and prevents intromission. In such cases lubrication of vulva and directing the penis in vulva may help. In stallion, due to premature full erection, the glans penis may become too large to enter vulva of small mare. In such cases vulvar lubrication, manually directing the penis, breeding the partners of suitable size and artificial insemination of the mare may be the possible solutions. Premature penile erection may prevent coitus in dog. Full penile erection does not take place until the dog penis is in the vagina of bitch. In such cases too, artificial breeding may be done.

Loss of sensory innervations of the glans penis

Loss of sensory innervations of the glans penis may be caused by trauma and this prevents natural intromission and thrust reflex necessary for ejaculation. Inexperienced males suffer more than the experienced male (that had earlier breeding).

Urinary caliculi

Urinary caliculi lodged in urethra may cause pain, obstruction, rupture, bleeding and deposition of semen at improper place in vagina. The caliculi may be removed surgically but urethral strictures, formation of other caliculi in the same area and formations of the adhesions are the common sequele following operation.

Pain yielding causes

Pain caused by infections of the genital organs including accessory sex glands, peritonitis, traumatic gastritis and cardiac diseases may cause refusal to copulate.

IMPOTENTIA GENERANDI (INCAPACITY OR REDUCED CAPACITY TO FERTILIZE IN MALES)

Impotentia generandi in males is characterized by normal sexual desire as well as normal ability to copulate but the fertility is either subnormal or absent. Impotentia generandi may be of following types :

A. Impotentia generandi associated with production of apparently normal semen. It may be due to either (a) infectious diseases or (b) inherited sperm defects.

B. Impotentia generandi associated with production of semen, which is abnormal in morphology, concentration, motility and other qualities.

A. Impiotentia generandi associated with apparently normal semen

(a) Infectious diseases

The semen ejaculates of the bulls infected with brucellosis, campylobacteriosis, trichomoniasis and IBR-IPV etc. may be normal in motility, concentration and morphology but such samples result in embryonic/foetal death, abortion, and signs of infertility.

(b) Inherited sperm defects

DIADEM EFFECT (EVERSION OF THE GALEA CAPITIS AND CRATER SHAPED DEPRESSIONS IN THE NUCLEUS; NUCLEAR POUCH FORMATION DEFECT)

The bulls with this type of inherited sperm abnormality are infertile or nearly sterile though the semen has normal motility and concentration of spermatozoa. This defect is a sign of severe disturbance in spermiogenesis. In this defect there are invaginations of the nuclear membrane and the defect is confined near the anterior border of the post-nuclear cap in the equatorial segment of the sperm head. Feulgen stain and phase contrast microscopy are helpful in revealing this defect.

KNOBBED SPERMATOZOA

This defect is an acrosomal defect and in this defect there is accentrically placed thickening of the acrosome. Knobbed spermatozoa is an inherited autosomal, recessive, sex linked defect related to defective spermiogenesis involving golgi apparatus. This defect has been noted in bulls, boars and dogs. The semen sample with knobbed spermatozoa have normal spermatozoa motility and concentration but are associated with infertility. Ordinary routine staining would not reveal this defect. The defect can be seen after staining with Eosin-B, Fast green or with phase contrast microscopy. Certain bulls may have as many as 50% or more knobbed spermatozoa. In this defect the sperm is incapable of penetrating and fertilizing the ovum.

GENE OR CHROMOSOMAL DEFECTS

Gene or chromosomal defects may occur at the time of meiosis resulting in infertility with semen appearing good to excellent. The decline in fertility is due to intrachromosomal aberrations. The electron microscopic study of the genital epithelium of the affected bulls show structural changes in the chromosomes including translocations and inversions. There may be fertilization but since the zygote lacks balanced gene complement, it dies in early gestation or if the defective chromosomal complement is brought to the next generation, nearly 50% of the male individuals are infertile. Greater the number of genes involved in translocation and inversion, greater are the chances of infertility/sterility.

ATYPICAL BASIC NUCLEAR PROTEINS

Atypical basic nuclear proteins may be formed due to defect in sperm cell chromatin which occur during spermiogenesis. The semen picture is revealed as normal. The atypical basic nuclear proteins possibly interfere with activation of ova and/or penetration of sperm into ova.

INHERENT ENZYMATIC DISTURBANCES

Impaired fertility may also be related to some inherent enzymatic disturbances that may cause early death of the spermatozoa in the female genital organs.

B. Impotentia generandi associated with apparently abnormal semen

This type of infertility may be associated with pathology of testes, epididymis, vas deferens, accessory sex glands, and urethra or may be associated with abnormal semen production due to congenital or hereditary causes or due to acquired causes.

CRYPTORCHIDISM

Normally the testes are situated in the scrotum at or soon after birth through descent of testes. Failure of one or both the testes to descend into scrotum at appropriate time is known as cryptorchidism. Unilateral cryptorchidism is more common and the affected males are near normally fertile because of normal production of semen from the testis located in the scrotum. Cryptorchidism, if bilateral, results in sterility. In retained or cryptorchid testes, spermatogenesis is inhibited because of elevated temperature of the affected testis Cryptorchid testis is usually small in size, soft and flaccid. The cryptorchidism is seen in all domestic species. It is most commonly seen in stallions, boars and dog, less commonly seen in rams and bucks, uncommonly seen in bull and rarely in cat. The cryptorchidism is a hereditary condition and such animal should not be used for breeding.

IMPERFECT DESCENT OF TESTIS

Sometimes in bull, the testes though not cryptorchid, are located fairly high in the scrotum and are somewhat horizontal. Such animals are called "high flankers". This may due to attachment of cremaster muscle to the caudal aspect of testis, fixation of the lower end of scrotum to the perineal region or lower attachment of gubernaculum. In such animals, because of imperfect thermoregulatory mechanisms, the testes show degeneration and atrophy and the fertility is impaired. The condition might be genetic in nature.

SCROTAL OR INGUINAL HERNIA

Scrotal or inguinal hernias are reported commonly in stallions and boars. A large scrotal hernia would greatly interfere with the testicular function of the affected side because of elevated temperature and increased pressure on testes caused by herniated loop of the intestine. In smaller degree of inguinal hernia, there are greater chances of strangulation of the intestine. If mating is allowed by the male, there are fair chances that due to increased abdominal pressure at coitus, the loop of the intestine may be forced trough inguinal opening and thus the condition may worsen. The condition is considered to be of hereditary in origin. Animals with inguinal hernia should be castrated and should not be used for breeding.

TESTICULAR HYPOPLASIA

The testicular hypoplasia is a unilateral or bilateral condition noted at the time of puberty or later. The condition is commonly noted in bulls, rams, boars and stallions. In bulls, the incidence is up to 23% of the testicular pathology cases. Testicular hypoplasia is a congenital and hereditary condition caused by single recessive autosomal gene with incomplete penetration. The condition is due to lack of or marked reduction in spermatogonia in the gonad during the fetal life. There may be (1) failure of germ cells to develop in the yolk sac, (2) failure of germ cells to migrate to the gonad, (3) failure of the germ cells to multiply in the gonad and (4) extensive degeneration of the germ cells after they have reached the gonads.

The **symptoms** vary greatly depending upon the degree of testicular hypoplasia. It may be from slight and often unsuspected hypoplasia to either unilateral or bilateral complete hypoplasia. Left side testicular hypoplasia is more common (66.7%) compared to right side testicular hypoplasia. Lowered conception rates are associated with bilateral testicular hypoplasia. Only in bilateral complete testicular hypoplasia, the animals are sterile. In most of the cases of testicular hypoplasia, the sexual desire is excellent and the coitus is prompt. The affected testes are reduced in size and are usually firmer. The affected bulls have small and firm epididymis indicating reduction in spermatogenesis as well as in gonadal sperm reserves. The semen picture is characterized by low concentration of spermatozoa, low motility, high incidence of proximal protoplasmic droplets and abnormal spermatozoa. In bilateral cases the semen is usually clear and watery with only few or no spermatozoa. Giant cells (or multinucleated cells with 6-8 nuclei) and medusa cells (or ciliated cells) from efferent tubules may be observed in the ejaculate. These multinucleated cells are the result of incomplete maturation division of the primary spermatocytes. The nuclei divide but the cytoplasmic divisions are not complete. The development of the other genital organs (except testes) is normal. Histologically the seminiferous tubules are very much underdeveloped with only the basal layer of the cells being present. Varying degree of spermatogenesis may be present from spermatogonia, spermatocytes and spermatids to abnormal and normal spermatozoa.

The **diagnosis** of testicular hypoplasia should not be done before two years of age in bulls and horses and before one year of age in boar, ram, dog and cat, unless the male is well grown. In young and immature bulls that are underdeveloped and are poorly fed, testicular hypoplasia may be erroneously diagnosed.

The **prognosis** in testicular hypoplasia is poor since the condition is hereditary. The affected animals should not be used for breeding purpose.

The **treatment** of testicular hypoplasia is not successful and the animals should be culled.

TESTICULAR DEGENERATION

It is estimated that 75 to 80 per cent of the testicular pathology is related to testicular degeneration. The epithelium of the testis is most sensitive to any adverse influence. Generalized disease processes bring about bilateral testicular degeneration and the local testicular lesions bring about unilateral testicular degeneration. The testicular degeneration is very rapid (may be within hours or days) but the testicular regeneration process is very slow and it may take several weeks to several months for recovery. Further when the basal layer of the germinal epithelium (including spermatogonia and Sertoli cells) is destroyed, regeneration is not possible and the animal becomes sterile. The changes in testicular degeneration are almost common in all species e.g. reduced concentration of spermatozoa, reduced motility of spermatozoa, increased number of abnormal spermatozoa, atrophic seminiferous tubules and testes smaller and softer. Such changes would depend upon the degree of degeneration. In chronic cases of testicular degeneration, the testis may become firm due to fibrosis and even there may be deposition of calcium in areas peripheral to the rete testis.

The **various causes** for testicular degeneration are :

1. **Thermal influence :** Prolonged elevated body temperature as in certain infectious diseases, prolonged high environmental temperature particularly associated with high humidity, direct heating of scrotum, increase in the scrotal temperature due to any other cause e.g. irritants, dermatitis, cryptorchidism and ectopic testes cause testicular degeneration. Summer infertility in exotic bulls and rams is a common phenomenon.

2. **Vascular lesions of the testes :** Interference in the blood circulation of the testes e.g. torsion of testes, presence of strongyle larvae in the testicular artery in the horse, varicoceles of the spermatic vein may cause infarction and may affect heat regulatory mechanism leading to degenerative changes in the testis.

3. **Irradiation :** Irradiation produces interference with spermatogenesis and spermatogonia, spermatids and spermatocytes are injured. The most sensitive are spermatocytes, while the Leydig cells and Sertoli cells are quite resistant to radiation. The first change is the increase in the number of abnormal spermatozoa and then there is decrease in the concentration of the spermatozoa.

4. **Hormonal causes :** Tumors of the anterior pituitary gland or hypothalamus interfere with the production of gonadotropic hormones. This is seen most commonly in dog and rarely in other animals. In dog these tumors are also associated with testicular atrophy and de-generation and with obesity and is referred to as *"dystrophia adiposogenitalis"*. Sertoli cell tumors produce excessive amount of estrogen. Leydig cell tumors produce excessive amount of testosterone and estrogen. These excessive steroids may suppress the production of FSH and may cause testicular degeneration.

5. **Age effects :** Old age has been reported to be associated with rather permanent and pro-gressive testicular degeneration nearly in all species of animals e.g. dogs over 10 years of age, cats over 12 years of age and bulls over 8-10 years of age. This phenomenon is affected by diseases, genetic and managemental factors.

6. **Trauma, stress or diseases :** Trauma, stress or disease factors may cause rapid testicular degeneration in males e.g. long duration shipping under stress of heat or cold, severe fatigue, traumatic gastritis, internal abscesses, severe and multiple contusions, severe arthritis, severe myiasis (disease of tissue or cavity by larvae and flies), laminitis, foot rot, traumatic lesions of testis and scrotum.

7. **Localized or systemic infectious diseases :** Localized or systemic infectious diseases are common causes of testicular degeneration. Infections causing orchitis or epididymitis as a normal inflammatory process produce heat, oedema and congestion etc. The thick and firm tunica albuginea restrict normal swelling of the testis and testicular degeneration occurs. Any disease localized in the testis may cause abscessation and testicular degeneration. Brucella abortus, Mycobacterium tuberculosis, Corynebacterium pyogenes, Actinomyces bovis, IBR-IPV virus, Epivag virus, Canine distemper virus etc. produce orchitis, epi-didymitis, testicular degeneration and testicular fibrosis. Severe obstructive lesions affecting the efferent ducts may cause back pressure resulting in testicular degeneration. Sporadic infections e.g. Streptococci, Staphylococci, E. coli, Proteus and Pseudomonas, all may cause orchitis in animals.

8. **Diseases causing fever, debilitation, inanition and loss of body weight :** Diseases causing fever, debilitation, inanition and loss of body weight etc. may cause testicular degeneration

(e.g. pneumonia, peritonitis, IBR-IPV infection, FMD, Johne's diseases, shipping fever, severe parasitism, chronic arthritis etc.) by direct heating effect, localized pressure, localized inflammatory reaction or by suppressing the release of gonadotropic hormones from the anterior pituitary gland. Diets sufficient for growth and maintenance of the body are also adequate for fertility.

9. **Nutrition :** Underfeeding and malnutrition producing debility and loss of body weight may suppress the release of gonadotropic hormones from the anterior pituitary gland and may produce testicular degeneration. Severe Vit. A deficiencies may produce testicular degeneration. High feeding levels and obesity generally do not affect the semen quality in normal males but it does effect willingness to mount.

10. **Poisons :** Various poisons may adversely affect the germinal epithelium. Dipping of rams in arsenic solutions causes degeneration of seminiferous tubules. Antimony compounds (for treating heartworms) in dog causes temporary infertility. Chlorinated napthalenes produce testicular degeneration in bulls and rams. Alkylating agents, Cadmium chloride and Amphotericin B produce testicular degeneration in a number of species.

11. **Autoimmunization :** Experimentally (not in natural cases) autoimmunization with s/c injections of autologous testicular material together with Freund's adjuvant has been reported to cause testicular degeneration.

12. **Testicular tumors :** Testicular tumors are not common in bulls and buffalo bulls and in these species only isolated cases of testicular neoplasms have been recorded. In dogs the testicular tumors are common. In other species the testicular tumors are unusual. The testicular tumors may originate from interstitial cells, Sertoli cells and from germinal epithelium. Usually the tumors are observed in old age. The large tumors may cause testicular degeneration either due to their compressing effect or due to excess of steroids produced by interstitial or Sertoli cell tumors.

The **signs** of testicular degeneration are almost similar in all species and may range from mild to severe depending upon the cause, duration and the degree of degeneration.

The testicular size is usually reduced because of the atrophy of the seminiferous tubules. In acute orchitis, inflammatory conditions, obstruction of the efferent tubules and testicular degeneration, the testicular size is usually increased.

The consistency of the testes is generally soft and yielding in testicular degeneration. Nearly 80% of the testes is composed of seminiferous tubules and their contents. In mild cases, consistency differs only slightly. In acute cases there is tense swelling and enlargement with pain and heat. The chronic cases may show fibrosis and calcification.

The sex drive is usually not affected except in painful conditions or in severely debilitating conditions (Leydig cells are more resistant to stress factors than the cells of germinal epithelium).

The *semen picture* is helpful in diagnosing testicular degeneration. It should be remembered that a wide period (60-70 days in bull, 40-45 days in stallion, 60-70 days in ram, 50-60 days in boar and 60-70 days in Dog) is required for spermatogenesis until sperms are ejaculated. Hence it is necessary to take several samples at weekly or greater intervals in diagnosing testicular degeneration. Moreover semen samples taken after a long period of sexual rest may be misleading as such samples, are of poor quality and have increased number of dead spermatozoa. The semen may be watery and translucent with azoospermia (no sperms) and oligozoospermia (reduced sperm concentration). The sperm motility is reduced because of increased percentage of abnormal cells,

Nomenclature in semen analysis

Parameter	Criterion	Nomenclature
Volume	No volume	Aspermia
	Reduced volume	Hypospermia
	Increased volume	Hyperspermia
Sperm concentration	Zero concentration	Azoospermia
	Normal concentration	Normozoospermia
	Reduced concentration	Oligozoospermia
	Increased concentration	Polyzoospermia
Sperm motility	Decreased motility	Asthenozoospermia
Sperm viability	All dead sperms	Necrozoospermia
Abnormal sperms	High percentage of abnormal sperm	Teratozoospermia

dead cells and poorly viable cells. There is an increase in abnormal heads, middle pieces and tails. The occurrence of large number of primary abnormality are more indicative of testicular degeneration (e.g. macrocephalic sperms, microcephalic sperms, short broad heads, elongated narrow heads, pear shaped heads, double heads, double middle pieces and tails, swelling of middle pieces, kinked or coiled middle pieces and tails and abaxially attached middle pieces). Giant or multi-nucleated cells are increased in testicular degeneration. The fertility may very from only slight reduction in conception rate to severe infertility.

The **prognosis** in testicular degeneration is variable depending upon the causative factor, duration and the degree of degeneration and the age of the animal. In young animals, in slight and mild cases and with transient and correctable causes, the prognosis is fair to good. The prognosis is poor in chronic cases, advanced testicular degeneration, severe orchitis, abscessation, and bilateral tumors and in cases with severe secondary lesions in the epididymis, accessory glands and vas deferens. Severe testicular degeneration leads to fibrosis and calcification and recovery is never possible.

The **treatment** of testicular degeneration consists of correction of the causative factor/alleviation of causative factor and sexual rest. Some mild cases can be treated. Some cases may require a balanced diet supplemented with Vit. A and quality proteins. Some exercise may be required in some cases. Air conditioning and cooling may be recommended for exotic bulls and rams in tropical climate. In cases of acute orchitis sexual rest and broad range antibiotics together with glucocorticoids may be given. Heat or counter irritants should not be used. Suitable cold packs may be applied. The use of hormones has not been found satisfactory. Testosterone, FSH preparations and Thyroxin have not been found to be of therapeutic value in cases of testicular degeneration and hypoplasia. Further, gonadotropic hormones need to be given for months and these should be derived from the same biological source to prevent developing of antihormones. If the orchitis is unilateral, affected testis may be removed to hasten recovery and to save breeding life of valuable animals. *Brucella*-infected bulls or boars should not be used in *Brucella*-free animals either naturally or artificially. Testes with the tumors should be removed to prevent secondary tumors due to metastases. Testicular tumors are common in cryptorchid testes and cryptorchid testes should be removed in the young age.

Some testosterone preparations and their doses in large animals		
Name of the drug	Manufacturer	Dose
1. Restore (Mesterolone) 25 mg tab.	Brown and Burk	2 tab. t.i.d. for 1 month followed by 2 tab. b.i.d. for 1 month
2. Sustanon 250	Infar	1 ml i/m every 1-2 weeks
3. Testanon 25 (Testosterone proprionate 25 mg/ml)	Infar	1 ml i/m every 2-3 days
4. Testoviron depot (250 mg)	German Remedies	250 mg i/m every 1-2 weeks followed by 250 mg i/m every 3-4 week
5. Aquaviron 25	Nicholas	1 ml i/m every 2-3 days

ORCHITIS

Orchitis denotes inflammation of the testis. It is caused mostly by bacterial infections (e.g. Brucella abortus) and by some viral agents (e.g. Epivag in African countries). It is generally haematogenous in origin. It may be caused from wounds penetrating the scrotal sac and several infectious agents may be involved in causing orchitis e.g. Streptococci, Staphylococci, C. pyogenes, Proteus, E. coli, P. aeruginosa etc. It may also be caused by descending infections from accessory sex glands through vas deferens.

In acute cases the scrotum becomes hot, painful and oedematous. There may be rise in body temperature and anorexia.

The treatment would consists of sexual rest, antiseptic dressing, application of ice packs and broad range antibiotics with glucocorticoids by parenteral routes. Brucella infected bulls should never be used on Brucella free herds either naturally or through artificial insemination.

TESTICULAR FIBROSIS

Testicular fibrosis is usually the end result of testicular inflammation and testicular degeneration. In testicular fibrosis the Leydig cells and seminiferous tubules are replaced by fibrous tissue. Some areas of necrosis, calcification and lymphocytic infiltration may also be seen. The ejaculates are watery and contain few or no sperms.

TESTICULAR CALCIFICATION

Testicular calcification is associated with testicular degeneration and is usually bilateral. In one study 9.55% incidence of testicular calcification was recorded in male buffalo genitals collected from abattoir. Such testes are hard.

TESTICULAR NEOPLASMS

These does not appear to be common in bulls and buffalo bulls. Testicular tumors are common in dogs. The testicular tumors originate from interstitial cells, Sertoli cells and germinal epithelium. Usually the testicular tumors are observed in old age. The large testicular tumors cause degeneration either due to their compressing effect or due to excess of steroid hormones produced by interstitial cell/Sertoli cell tumors.

EPIDIDYMITIS

Epididymitis is the inflammation of the epididymis. It is usually secondary to orchitis. The organisms cause perivascular lesions with oedema and fibrosis, resulting in epididymal obstruction, stasis of epididymal contents and extravasation (flowing out fluid from vessel) of semen. The high lipid and mycolic acid contents lead to the formation of spermatic granuloma.

The **diagnosis** is based on clinical palpation of the epididymis to detect enlargement, induration and spermatic granuloma. These lesions are observed in the tail region of the epididymis.

The **prognosis** is severe or poor even in moderate cases of epididymitis, because obstructions prevent discharge of spermatozoa from testes.

In valuable animals with unilateral epididymitis, unilateral castration may be performed provided accessory glands and vas deferens have no lesions. Such animals may be given long sexual rest.

SPERMIOSTASIS

Spermiostasis may be caused by blind rudimentary mesonephric tubules or ductuli aberrantes. These are most often defective efferent tubules. These defective tubules are attached to rete or epididymis and produce lesions mainly in the head of the epididymis. Other portions of the epididymis are only rarely involved. The condition is common in bucks and rams, less common in bulls and rare in other domestic animals. The condition is probably genetic in origin.

There is no treatment for this condition and because of hereditary nature of this condition, the affected animals should be culled.

TUMORS OF EPIDIDYMIS

Primary tumors of epididymis are rare in all animals. Testicular tumors, which are common in dog, may invade epididymis. Occasionally metastatic tumors may develop in the epididymis.

SEGMENTAL APLASIA OF THE MESONEPHRIC DUCT

Segmental aplasia of the mesonephric duct is a congenital hereditary condition and seen most commonly in bulls. The body and tail or all the epididymis and even the part of the vas deferens may be missing. In majority of the cases, the conditions is unilateral and the bull is fertile. The bilateral cases are sterile and the semen is watery with no sperm. There is no treatment and the affected animals should not be used in breeding programmes as the condition is hereditary.

PATHOLOGY OF THE VAS DEFERENS AND AMPULLA

Infections and inflammations of the vas deferens are usually associated with orchitis, epididymitis or seminal vesiculitis. Usually the infections are unilateral but may be bilateral. Several infectious organisms e.g. Brucella abortus, Streptococci, C. pyogenes and others including viruses may be responsible for this conditions.

Ampullitis is revealed as thickened, firm and painful enlargement. In ampullitis the semen contains pus cells and the motility of the spermatozoa is poor. If the motility is good after ejaculation, it would be lost rapidly on storage of semen.

SEMINAL VESICULITIS

Inflammations of the vesicular glands, which lie just lateral to the ampullae of the vas deferens are commonly seen. Their normal consistency is meaty and yielding and the lobulations are very clearly felt in normal condition.

The **incidence** has been reported varying from 3 to 4 percent in European breeds. Some cases are also reported in India.

Seminal vesiculitis **may be caused** by a variety of organisms including specific pathogens (like Brucella organisms, Mycobacterium bovis, Mycobacterium paratuberculosis, Chlamydia, Mycoplasma and certain viruses) and nonspecific opportunistic pathogens (like Streptococci, Staphylococci, Actinobacilli, Corynebacteria etc.). The organisms may localize in the seminal vesicle from other infected foci like rumenitis, liver abscesses and traumatic gastritis. Infections in the seminal vesicle may also come as an ascending infection (e.g. from prepuce) or as a descending infections (e.g. from infected ampulla, epididymis, vas deferens and testicle). In countries where brucellosis is present, Brucella abortus is the most common cause for seminal vesiculitis.

The seminal vesiculitis may be acute or chronic. In acute seminar vesiculitis there would be **signs** of localized peritonitis. Affected gland(s) may be enlarged and firm and there is pain on palpation. Purulent exudate is present in the semen consistently. Chronic seminal vesiculitis may or may not follow acute phase. There would be enlargement, fibrosis and loss of lobulations form the gland. Pain on palpation is usually absent. In both the forms, semen of affected bulls contains purulent material, leukocytes and epithelial cells and the motility of the sperms is decreased.

The **prognosis** in seminal vesiculitis may be fair to poor depending upon duration and severity of the infection, nature of infection and the presence of other infected foci. In some young bulls recovery may be spontaneous but in older bulls affected with chronic seminal vesiculitis, the cure is rare. Males affected with brucellosis, tuberculosis mycoplasmosis and with lesions of testes, epididymides, ampullae or prostate should be slaughtered.

In some younger bulls **treatment** with broad range antibiotics sensitive to causative agent for 2-3 weeks, removing the contents by massage may cause recovery. The culture of the semen is not satisfactory because of the contamination from sheath. Acute cases generally become chronic and chronic cases generally become fibrotic. In certain cases where lesions are detected extensively in seminal vesicle, adhesions are extensive and conservative treatment is not deemed fit, the affected vesicular gland may be removed surgically.

PROSTATITIS

Prostatitis is uncommon in animals except in dog. In bulls inflammatory processes of prostate gland have been found at necropsy but not clinically. Prostatitis in dog above 5 years of age is common and often associated with hyperplasia of the gland. It may occur as ascending or descending infections or from haematogenous infections. Several organisms may be responsible for this conditions and among which Brucella canis, E. coli, Streptococci and Proteus are most common. The condition may be diffused or local. Leukocytes are frequently found in urine and at prepucial orifice. Prostatitis in dogs may be present without causing any abnormal sign evident to the owner. In acute phase there may be pain and the condition may be characterized by arched back, stiff gait in rear limbs, elevated temperature, elevated pulse rate, constipation and occasionally anorexia and vomiting. The cases of prostatitis frequently respond to broad range antibiotic treatment for prolonged period. In some cases that fail to respond to the ordinary antibiotics, a cultural sensitivity examination of the prostatic secretion may be made to determine antibiotic of choice. prostatitis due to Brucella canis does not respond to treatment.

PROSTATIC HYPERPLASIA

Prostatic hyperplasia is reported in dogs above 5 years of age that have not been castrated. The condition is probably due to an altered androgen-estrogen ratio with an excess of testosterone secreted causing hyperplasia of the prostate gland. Most of the times the prostatic hyperplasia would not show signs of illness and the dog is active and alert. The enlarged gland may contain small cysts. Cysts wall may be calcified. Prostatic caliculi are very rare. Dogs with prostatic hyperplasia are usually constipated.

Examination for **diagnosis** of prostatic hyperplasia in dog may be done bimanually per rectum and by abdominal palpation. Applying pressure on abdominal wall to the pelvic brim pushes the prostate caudally and this helps prostate palpation per rectum. The size, location and contour of the postate can also be evaluated by caudal abdominal radiography. Aspiration biopsy using a long needle is generally avoided since in cases with abscessation numerous bacteria may be seeded in the needle tract.

The most effective **treatment** for prostatic enlargement is castration. With castration involution of prostate begins within days and within 6-8 weeks the prostate is atrophied. Castration would not be effective to reduce cysts, abscesses or caliculi, if present. If castration is not feasible, estrogen therapy may be given. Estrogens are not antiandrogens. Estrogens suppress the production of pituitary gonadotropins, which cause atrophy of Leydig cells, and thus suppression of testosterone production. Diethylstilbestrol orally @ 1 mg per day for 5 days or Estradiol cypionate @ 0.1 mg per kg with maximum dose of 2 mg may be given intramuscularly. High prolonged dosing with estrogens may cause bone narrow depression with resultant aplastic anemia and leucopenia.

INHERITED OR CONGENITAL SPERM CELL DEFECTS

Inherited or congenital sperm cell defects are reported in male domestic animals in which male produces large number of the spermatozoa with similar defects.

Diadem effect (Nuclear pouch formation defect) : This defect is confined to the anterior border of the postnuclear cap and results from invaginations of the nuclear membrane. This defect is a sign of disturbed spermatogenesis. Feulgen stain and phase contrast microscopy would reveal this defect.

Knobbed sperm : This defect is noted in bulls and also in boars and dogs. This is an inherited autosomal recessive sex linked defect related to defective spermiogenesis involving the golgi apparatus. In this defect there is accentrically placed thickening of the acrosome. The defect is present in nearly 50% or more spermatozoa and the bulls are sterile. Special staining techniques are only helpful in diagnosing this defect. The defect can be seen after staining with Eosin B or Fast green or with phase contrast microscopy. In this defect the sperm is incapable of penetrating and fertilizing the ovum.

Decapitated sperm : This defect is associated with an ultrastructural abnormality in the neck or implantation region of the spermatozoa. The sperms, due to this ultra- structural abnormality in the neck region, disintegrate into heads and tails in the caput (head) epididymis.

Sterilizing tail stump : In this defect, instead of actual tail, there is a short tail stump (2-3 µ long).

Dag defect : In this defect of spermatozoa in bulls, the main piece is strongly coiled over the mid piece giving an impression of short tail. The defect is noted in about 40% of the spermatozoa. There is no evidence of any abnormality of the seminiferous tubules. The fibers in the axial filament were normal in the testes but abnormal when the cells reach the cauda (tail) epididymis. This defect is found associated with elevated levels of zinc in the spermatozoa as well as in seminal plasma. Such bulls have normal volume and sperm concentration in semen but the motility is only 10-20%. Such bulls are invariably infertile/sterile.

Pseudo droplet defect : In this defect 7-25% of the spermatozoa have rounded or elongated thickening on the mid piece. Reduced semen motility and infertility increases with age.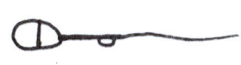

Cork screw defect : In this defect mid piece of the 10-15% spermatozoa is in the shape of a corkscrew. This is due to an irregular distribution of the mitochondrial sheath.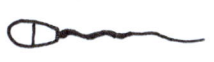

Returned tail and narrow head : The defect is noted in some families of Jersey breed. The defect is apparently genetic.

Inbreeding : Inbreeding generally results in reduced fertility accompanied by increase in the number of abnormal seminiferous tubules, poor semen quality and testicular hypoplasia. The fertility in between inbred lines differs widely, some with excellent fertility, some with poor fertility and some inbred lines may even vanish because of infertility.

Infertility in hybrids : When there are major differences in the number of chromosomes of the parents, infertility usually results. Sterility is more common in male hybrids. The examples of hybrid infertility are :

1. Horse (64) and ass (62) crosses Producing mule (sterile)
2. Goat (60) and sheep (54) crosses Conception occurs but all the embryos die
3. Bison (60) and domestic cattle (60) crosses Bulls are sterile
4. Yalk (60) and domestic cattle (60) crosses Bulls are sterile
5. Yalk (60) and zebu (60) crosses Bulls are sterile

Note : Within parentheses are (2n) chromosome numbers.

The inheritance of small and thick scrotum from the bison and yak causes an elevated scrotal temperature that affects the normal functioning of the seminiferous tubules due to poor thermo-regulation.

Intersex : Intersexes are invariably sterile. An intersex is an animal with congenital mal-formations of sexual development. Intersexes are broadly divided into 3 groups : (1) True herma-phrodites, (2) Male and female pseudohermaphrodites and (3) Freemartins. True hermaphrodites have various combinations of ovaries, testis and ovo-testes together with varying of bisexuality in accessory sex organs. In pseudohermaphrodites there exits discrepancy between the external genitalia and the gonad. Male pseudohermaphrodites have testes but female externalia. Female pseudo-hermaphrodites have ovaries and male externalia. Pseudohermaphrodites are more common than true hermaphrodites. Freemartin (in bovine) results from sexual modification of female twin due to exchange of blood from male twin in the uterus.

Cryptorchidism (incomplete decent of testis) : Cryptorchidism, if bilateral results in sterility. Unilateral cryptorchidism is more common and does not interfere much with fertility, as there is normal production of sperms from descended testis located in the scrotum. Cryptorchid testis is usually smaller in size and do not produce spermatozoa because, the spermatogenesis is inhibited due to elevated temperature. Cryptorchidism is seen in all species. It is more common in stallions, boars and dogs. In rams and bucks it is less common. The condition is uncommon in bulls and rare in cats. The treatment of this condition in animals used for breeding should be discouraged.

Torsion or rotation of descended testis : Torsion or rotation of the descended testis is commonly observed in stallions and dogs and rarely in boars. The defect is congenital. The testicles are rotated and are held somewhat high in the scrotum. In normal stallions the tail of the epididymis is caudal but in this condition the tail of the epididymis is lateral. The testis is freely moveable in the scrotum. Usually the semen characteristics are not affected by this condition. In some stallions hiking of the leg on affected testis may cause congestion, swelling and pain and this may affect spermatozoa production from the affected testis.

Imperfect descent of testes : Sometimes in bulls due to the attachment of cremaster muscle to the caudal aspect of the testis and/or fixation of the distal end of the scrotum to perineal region, the testes may be located fairly high in position and horizontally. Such animals are called "high flankers". Thus the thermoregulatory mechanism of the testis does not function properly and as a result there is degeneration and atrophy of the testicular tissue along with impaired fertility. The condition may be genetic in nature.

Scrotal or inguinal hernias : Scrotal or inguinal hernia is common in stallions and boars, less common in bulls, dogs and rams and is rare in cats. The condition in hereditary. A large hernia interfere with normal thermoregulatory function of the scrotum and testis of the affected side because of high temperature and high pressure caused by herniated intestinal loop. In inguinal hernia, there are greater chances of strangulation of intestine. The animals with inguinal hernia should not be allowed for breeding. If mating is allowed, there are chances that due to increased abdominal pressure at coitus, the loop of the intestine may be further forced through inguinal opening and thus the condition may further worsen.

MISCELLANEOUS DISEASES AFFECTING THE REPRODUCTIVE FUNCTIONS

Sometimes failure of proper delivery of semen may lead to infertility/sterility. In some animals glans penis may have fistulous opening of urethra ventrally and in such cases, semen is deposited in the middle of vagina instead of cranial portion or over the cervical oss. In rams necrosis of urethral process or lodging of caliculi in urethral process may also lead to similar situation.

Some bulls have high fertility and some low fertility and the cause remains unexplained. Fertility is determined also genetically. The semen of some bulls do not withstand freezing. The fertility of bulls also varies from herd to herd.

Chapter 7

Introduction, Development, History, Advantages and Disadvantages of A.I.

Till date artificial insemination (A.I.) is the single technique that has been most popular in veterinary practice and has been universally accepted for the genetic improvement of the animals. This technique has brought tremendous improvement in the milk production through wide use of highly selected sires having high genetic potential for milk production in thousands of inferior cows with low milk production. This technique has been widely accepted in cattle. Other species like buffalo, sheep, goat, swine, horse and dog are also covered by A.I. but not so extensively. The earliest documented use of A.I. technique appears in 1780 when Lazzaro Spallanzani, an Italian physiologist artificially inseminated a bitch which gave birth to 3 pups. A.I. as a technique for breeding was developed and revolutionized in Russia around 1900 by Ivanoff. Shortly, thereafter, A.I. technique was adopted in farm animals in Japan. In India, A.I. technique was used in 1939 by Kumaran (as claimed by him) at Palace Dairy Farm, Mysore. A.I. was first started at I.V.R.I. Izatnagar in the year 1942 in cattle as well as in buffalo. The results of A.I. at five regional research stations namely, Montgomery (now in Pakistan), Izatnagar, Patna, Calcutta and Bangalore were highly encouraging and opened doors for livestock improvement in India through this technique.

ADVANTAGES OF A.I.

1. Maximum utilization of sire

Several insemination doses are prepared from one ejaculate and thus proven sires are utilized to their maximum. Through the use of A.I., a single bull in its life-time may easily cover up to 1 lac female cattle.

2. Economical technique

In A.I. programmes only selected bulls are kept for breeding purpose. This reduces work load and expenditure on bulls.

3. Herd improvement

The use of selected proven sires through A.I. brings about genetic improvement in the herd.

4. Better safety

Since only selected bulls are kept in A.I. programmes, the dangers are minimized. Further, since males are not brought to the farm or females, it further leads to better safety.

5. Reduced risk of venereal diseases

Bulls kept for A.I. purpose are regularily examined for their general as well as reproductive health. Diseased bulls are either properly treated or culled. This reduces risk of spreading sexually transmitted diseases.

6. Overcoming different sizes of two partners

Great variations in the size of male and female partners may prevent natural mating. Cow with either extremely large or extremely small size may be covered through A.I. without any difficulty.

7. Overcoming physical inability

The bulls which for some reason or other are unable to copulate, may be utilized in artificial insemination (e.g. from such bull semen may be collected using electro-ejaculator).

8. Covering cows that refuse mounting

Some females which are in good heat, but for some reason or the other refuse to be mounted, may be bred through A.I.

9. Early detection of diseases

Since during semen collection or during artificial insemination, the genitalia of both males and females are closely approached and inspected, the genital defects are easily noted, which otherwise may remain undetected for longer period of time.

10. Low transportation cost

Through the export/import of semen, international transportation cost is reduced which otherwise would greatly exceed to actual transportation of the animals.

11. Utilizing germplasm of dead animals

The deep freezed semen of the bull, which has died, may be utilized in artificial insemination programme.

12. Essential after estrus synchronization

Artificial insemination is almost essential for inseminating females after synchronization of estrus in large group of animals.

13. Better records

A.I. results in better record keeping.

14. Interesting technique

A.I. Stimulates greater interests in livestock breeding and also in better livestock management.

15. Valuable method in dog breeding under certain conditions

In dog, when mating is not possible, either due to timid nature or due to premature erection or due to unacquaintance of partners, artificial insemination technique may be of great value.

16. Helps selecting progeny tested proven sires

Because of wide use of extended semen/stored semen, the sire's daughters can be evaluated in more number and in minimum possible period. This is of great help in selecting progeny tested proven sires.

DISADVANTAGES OF A.I.

1. Fast spread of genetic abnormalities

Genetic abnormalities, if spread, spread at a very fast rate in artificial insemination programme. e.g. cystic ovary, poor conformation and lack of libido etc.

2. Loss of embryo/foetus with improper A.I.

Intrauterine inseminations of pregnant females may result into abortion.

3. Wanting skilled persons

For operations like semen collection, semen examination, semen extension, semen freezing and insemination, trained persons are required. Inseminators if not, careful would spread infections from animal to animal and from herd to herd.

4. Requiring special facilities

Artificial insemination requires special facilities like lab and equipments etc.

Chapter 8

Methods of Semen Collection in Various Species

1. SEMEN COLLECTION IN BULLS

The semen collection in **bulls** has been described in detail in Chapter 14.

2. SEMEN COLLECTION IN RAMS AND BUCKS

The semen from rams and bucks may be collected by the following 3 methods :

1. By collecting semen from the vagina of ewe following service.
2. By using artificial vagina.
3. By electro-ejaculation.

For collecting semen from vagina of ewe following service, the rams are trained to mount an anoestrous ewe. The vagina of the ewe is properly cleaned to remove mucus etc, prior to allowing service by the ram. If the ram refuses to serve the anoestrous ewe, an ewe in estrum may be used. After the service the semen is aspiratad from the vagina using a glass collecting piplte attached to a rubber bulb for suction. A pipelte attached to a syringe with rubber joint (as used in AI of cows with liquid semen) may also be used for collecting semen from vagina of the ewe. Since the semen collected by this method is usually contaminated, it is alway unsafe to use.

The artificial vagina for collecting semen from rams is similar to that used for collecting semen from bulls, but it is smaller. The hard rubber cylinder is about 20 cm long and 5 cm wide and the inner rubber liner is about 25 cm long and 3.75 cm wide. The A.V. is prepared in the same way as for bull. The temperature of the A.V. is critical and it should be at 45 to 50 C at the time of semen collection. The inner wall of the rubber liner is slightly lubricated with sterile lubricating jelly which is non-toxic to sperm cells. Air is inflated through valve until the inside lumen of the A.V. is occluded to a point when only one fingure can be inserted. Rams may be easily trained for semen collection using ewe in estrum. Subsequently any ewe or even artificial dummy may be used. In case of semen collcetion from **bucks**, an estrual doe is the most optimal mount animal.

Nonestrual doe generally creates problem by making lateral movements. Mounting and copulation in ram is very rapid and the operator should remain alert. The penis should not be touched with hand. The penis should be directed towards the artificial vagina by grasping sheath only.

The semen can also be collected from ram using **Electro-ejaculator**. With this equipment the semen may be collected from rams in standing position. Sometimes it may be necessary to restrain ram on its side with legs extended. Before inserting probe of suitable size, the rectum of ram/buck should be emptied using warm water anema. Gradually increasing electric current stimulations (2,5 and 8 volt peaks) are given with the current on for 2 to 5 seconds and off for 2-3 seconds. The penis should be held with gauze and the urethral process be directed into collection vial/tube to avoid ejaculation into the sheath. The semen samples collected by electro-ejaculation may occasionally be contaminated with urine. As with bull, the sperm concentration is usually less and ejaculate volume usually more by electro-ejaculation technique compared to semen collection either naturally or using artificial vagina.

3. SEMEN COLLECTION IN BOAR

In boars the collection period is long. It may take as long as five minutes or more during natural service. The semen from boars may be collected by the following 2 methods.

1. Gloved hand method and

2. Using artificial vagina

Pressure is more important for collecting semen from boars. Boar ejaculates, when the spiral tip of the penis is firmly engaged in sow's cervix or in artificial vagina or in operator's hand. Pressure should remain continuously exterted on spiral end of the penis for collection of semen from boars using either gloved hand method or using artificial vagina. The boar ejaculate consists of 3 fractions; presperm fraction, sperm-rich fraction, and post-sperm fraction. The first fraction (presperm fraction) contains seminal fluid, which has high bacterial count and also gelatinous material from Cowper's gland. In natural service this gelatinous material seals the cervix and prevents loss of semen. In collecting semen artificially the presperm fraction is discarded before collecting sperm rich fraction. Usually the boar emits only one sperm rich fraction but some boars may emit 2 or 3 sperm rich fractions interrupted in between by seminal fluid discharge. The sperm rich fraction is followed by post sperm fraction, which also contains about 20% of the gelatinous material.

In the **gloved hand method,** the boar is allowed to mount on estrous female or phantom. The operator stands on right side of the dummy. As the boar mounts and protrudes the penis, the operator catches twisted glans penis in gloved hand and exerts pressure on it so as to stimulate ejaculation. Relaxation of pressure would result in interruption of ejaculation. Once ejaculation starts and pressure is maintained the boar usually remains quiet until ejaculation is complete. The semen is collected in sterilized wide mouth bottle fitted with gauze filter.

Artificial vagina of various designs are developed to collect semen from boars. It is necessary that optimum pressure must be provided to the spirally twisted cranial portion of the penis so that it locks at complete erection as happens in natural service where it is almost fastened in the anterior vagina and cervical folds of the sow. Artificial vagina with a hard rubber cylinder of 12.5 cm length and 4.5 cm diameter with a rubber liner of 40 cm length and 3-3.5 cm diameter may be utilized for semen collection from boars. Small pieces of sponge rubber placed in between hard rubber cylinder and inner rubber lining where hot water at 45 to 50°C is placed, put increased pressure on penis. As the penis passes through the A.V., pressure is applied to the spirally twisted cranial end of the penis by the hand of the operator. The moderate pressure with fingures is kept continuous. Ejaculate once commenced, continues for 15 minutes of so. The ejaculate is collected is a plastic bottle or bag of 500 ml capacity that is in a cup or thermos of warm water at 39 C.

4. SEMEN COLLECTION IN STALLION

The ideal method for collection of semen from stallion is **by artificial vagina**. The A.V. for stallions is comparatively much larger to accommodate large, vascular and muscular penis when in erected position. Because of large size, comparatively heavier weight and vigorous thrust by stallion at ejaculation, the A.V. for stallions may also have a handle so that it is held firmly. The semen can be collected by using either phantom mare or estrous mare. If an estrous mare is used, her tail should be bandaged, perineal area should be thoroughly washed and cleaned and the mare should be properly hobbled. The operator should take all necessary precautions to protect himself/herself from injuries from mare and as well as from stallion. Use of helmets during artificial collection of semen from stallion is an added precaution. The mare or phantom should be of appropriate height. Before ejaculation the stallion's penis should be properly washed with mild soap solutions and then rinsed with clean water to remove smegma and other debris.

The A.V. is prepared by filling it with hot water to obtain temperature and proper pressure. The optimum internal temperature of the A.V. is 45 to 50°C. Higher temperatures would cause irritation to stallion's penis and may also damage sperms. The pressure inside A.V. should be such that the stallion should be able to penetrate the penis in adequately lubricated artificial vagina. Collection bottles are warmed to body temperature and are attached to A.V. just before collection. The optimum temperature and pressure, together with friction stimulates the stallion to ejaculate. Pulsation at the base of the penis is the characteristic for ejaculation. Ejaculation is completed in about 15 to 20 seconds. Gel from collected semen should be removed by careful aspiration using a syringe.

5. SEMEN COLLECTION FROM DOG

The semen from dog may be obtained by the following methods :
1. Manual manipulation
2. By artificial vagina

Manual manipulation is the simplest and cheapest method of semen collection in dogs. An estrous bitch is exposed to the dog. When the dog shows sexual interests in bitch, about 3-4 cm penis of the dog is exposed by pushing the prepucial skin caudally. The base of the penis behind the bulbus glandis is grasped and applied moderate pressure with fingures. Masturbation may also be helpful. Some dogs may be trained to ejaculate semen even in the absence of a teaser bitch, but in such cases sperm cell concentration is usually low. The semen is collected using a glass/plastic funnel attached to a warm tube into a warm vial or a barrel of syringe secured to prevent semen leakage. Maintaining proper pressure behind bulbus glandis is important for collecting sufficient semen. Ejaculation may last for 10-15 minutes. The first portion of the ejaculate contains few sperm cells. The sperm rich portion of the ejaculate is whitish-grey-milky.

The semen from dogs can also be collected using **Artificial Vagina**. The artificial vagina for dog is usually 19-20 cm in length and about 5 cm in diameter. The temperature of the artificial vagina should be around 40-42°C and lubrication is not needed. As far as possible, do not allow the dog to urinate and mark the area. This act of dog would result in urine in the ejaculate. In case the dog urinates and marks the area, a few drops of semen may be discarded on the ground in order to clean the passage of urethra of the urine residue. The dogs penis is stimulated through prepucial sheath by manipulation. When the erected penis is out, A.V. is slipped over it. In long haired breeds it should be ensured that no hair comes in between the penis and the artificial vagina. After semen collection, the artificial vagina is gently removed because the dog's penis remains engorged. If the A.V. is not removed in a gentle way there may be damage to the superficial vessels, which may be painful and may even cause infection and lack of libido subsequently.

Chapter 9

A.I. Techinques

The techniques of A.I. using chilled and frozen semen in **cattle** are described in Chapter 18 (Fig. 18.1).

Artificial insemination in **buffalo** is done by recto-vaginal technique similar to that of cows. Buffaloes, when manipulated per rectum bleed easily. All precautions should be taken to prevent straining and bleeding.

For insemination, the **ewe** is restrained in a crate that holds her securely and limits her movement making the examination and insemination easier for the operator. Holding the ewe by helper with its rear elevated greatly helps in artificial insemination. The small-sized speculum, lubricated with liquid paraffin is inserted in the ewe's vagina. 0.5 to 1.0 ml of semen is drawn into pipette attached to a syringe with rubber joint. Some amount of air behind semen helps in complete expulsion of semen from the catheter. By means of a light source the cervix is located and the tip of the inseminating catheter is inserted into the cervical canal and the semen is deposited.

For insemination, the **sow** is put in crate to minimize movement. The vulva is washed and wiped with clean tissue paper/absorbent cotton/towel. Various types of catheters for A.I. in swine are designed to facilitate deposition of semen into the uterus. All types of inseminating catheters are inserted dorsocranially to avoid entering the urethra. It is very important to avoid the entry of the catheter into the urethral opening, which is located ventrally in the posterior part of the vagina. The catheter is passed through the cervix to reach the uterus. Resistance in passing the catheter is overcome by rotating the catheter counterclockwise. Large volume (50-100 ml) of extended semen (having 10 billion sperms) in plastic bottle or bag is gently deposited into the cervix and uterus of the sow over a period of 3-5 minutes.

For insemination, the **mare** should be suitably restrained. Mare's tail should be bandaged with sterile gauze or bandage. The external genitalia, perineal region and buttocks should be thoroughly washed with soap and water, rinsed with clean water and wiped. The catheter is passed in vagina along with the hand encased in a sterile sleeve or disposable glove. The index fingure in the cervix assists in guiding the catheter. The amount of extended semen should be 10 to 40 ml depending upon the size of the mare. Mare is inseminated on second to fourth day and if the mare is still in heat, insemination is repeated on fifth and sixth day. Mares should be inseminated with minimum of 100-200 millions normal motile sperms. The recommendations vary up to 500 million normal motile sperms. The semen is deposited in the uterus. Spermatozoa retain their fertilizing capacity for 4-6 day in mare's reproductive tract. Air should be prevented from entering the vagina after insemination during the course of withdrawing hand from the vagina.

The insemination in **bitches** should be performed 2 to 3 days after the onset of true estrus (i.e. when the bitch allows mounting) or 10-12 days after onset of post estrous bleeding. Second insemination may be given after 1 to 2 day. Ovulation in bitch occurs 1 to 2 days after the onset of true estrum, but the ova requires several days to cast off their polar bodies and to mature. Spermatozoa survive for 4-6 days or even more in the genital tract of bitch. A sterile plastic inseminating tube of about 20 cm (half the length of the catheter used for inseminating cows) fixed to a glass syringe and semen drawn in it may be used. The bitch should be placed on table at proper height and should be held securely by assistant. The presence of the owner may be helpful. The external genitalia are properly washed and dried. Lubricated vaginal speculum and light may be of help in locating the cervix. Inseminating pipette is introduced through the cervix. 5 to 10 ml of the extended semen with 200 million actively motile spermatozoa are deposited. The catheter may be inserted without the help of speculum. In this method, the inseminating catheter is passed between the vulvar lips, directing dorsally until it passes vestibule. The inseminating pipette is then directed horizontally and pushed towards or into the cervix. To prevent possible loss of semen, the rear of the bitch may be kept elevated for 3-5 minutes. Feathering of dorsal vaginal wall with fingure (in a clean and hygienic way) appears promoting passage of semen into the uterus. Insemination directly in the uterus of bitch appears impossible.

Chapter 10

Factors Affecting Semen Production

The spermatogenesis is a continuous process in most of the domestic animals. However, various factors affect both quality and quantity of the semen in animals. The various factors which affect semen production (both quality and quantity) are :

1. Genetic
2. Season
3. Transportation
4. Exercise
5. Diseases and
6. Nutrition

Genetic factors : Inherited genetic factors have been found associated with poor serving ability, poor fertility and poor libido. Inbreeding has detrimental effect on male's fertility. Heterosis is associated with better fertility in males. Certain specific morphological sperm defects have been reported to be inherited (e.g. diadem effect, knobbed spermatozoa, decapitated sperms, sterilizing tail stump, corkscrew middle piece, narrow head and returned tail, defective nuclear proteins in the spermatozoa and certain enzymatic disturbances). These defects may affect sperm motility, activation of ova, penetration of sperm in ova and early death of sperms in the female genital tract. These defects have been described under male's infertility.

Season : The semen quality varies with seasonal variations in temperature, humidity, solar radiation and convectional currents of the air. These seasonal factors may affect the testes directly or indirectly through neuroendocrine signals. In general male reproductive functions are depressed by high temperature, especially if, this is accompanied by high humidity. The duration of day light hours and temperature are also correlated with the quality of semen produced and its fertility. In heavy rain fall coastal areas, where humidity is 80-100% during monsoon, the breeding bulls show poor sex drive and poor semen quality. Exotic bulls do not perform well in high temperature climate and this heat stress deteriorates semen quality. Spermatogonia are least affected by heat stress but spermatocytes, spermatids and spermatozoa are affected more by heat stress. Leydig cells are generally not affected by high heat. The semen quality of buffalo bulls generally remains good in spring season and fairly good in winter season. During summer and autumn there is decline in quality of semen in buffalo bulls. Buffalo bulls are more sensitive to heat and cold compared to cattle bulls. The buffalo bulls have less efficient thermoregulatory mechanism and thus have wide variation in semen quality in different seasons. The percentage of normal sperms in Romney Marsh rams brought in U.P. for improving indigenous breeds of sheep declined from 96.2% in January to 72.5% in February. The wave motion of semen was almost absent in June. During the months from July to September spermatogenic activity was almost ceased. The restoration of the spermatogenic activity started from end of October. In the month of November about 90% of the Spermatozoa were normal. The semen quality remained excellent during the months of December and January. During the summer and autumn, the semen quality deteriorates also in bucks. Severe chilling would also result in unsatisfactory ejaculates and bulls exposed to severe cold should be provided with thick and dry bedding.

Transportation : Short distance transportation does not affect the semen quality much. Long distance transportation of breeding bulls may temporarily deteriorate semen quality. Long distance transport of breeding bulls may cause increased steroid excretion in urine, which may subsequently be followed by decreased libido and morphological abnormalities of spermatozoa in semen. The transportation stress deteriorates the semen quality only temporarily. The semen quality improves with the alleviation of the transportation stress.

Exercise : Regular exercise keeps the bull alert and in good physical condition. There was no difference in the quality of semen in between bulls receiving 1 hour or 2 hours exercise per day. Exercise just before semen collection would usually cause decline in the ejaculate volume.

Diseases : Diseases causing high fever temporarily deteriorate semen quality. Diseases causing debility and inanition, may suppress the production of gonadotropins and this may cause atrophy and degeneration of seminiferous tubules. Senile changes are also associated with testicular atrophy and degeneration. Diseases of scrotum, testicles, other male duct system and of accessory sex glands are likely to adversely affect the quality and quantity of the ejaculate.

Nutrition : The qualitative and quantitative nutritional requirements for optimum reproduction in males do not exceed than those required for their growth/maintenance. The ration should be well balanced in carbohydrate, proteins, minerals and vitamins. The deficiency of a single nutrient is generally not noted but rather the deficiencies are usually of multiple type. Prolonged nutritional deficiencies of protein, carbohydrate, Vit. A and trace minerals may adversely affect semen production. Low plane of nutrition causes delay in puberty and sexual maturity. Severe nutritional deficiencies for prolonged period would cause loss of physical condition, atrophy of testes, loss of sexual desire and less ejaculate volume with less spermatozoa. High plane of nutrition has not been found to have convincing effect on semen production. However, overfed males are obese and lazy and are reluctant to readily ejaculate semen. Such lazy bulls frequently develop weakness in legs. Fat may also develop around testes especially in the dorsal part in overfed and fat bulls. The fat, if accumulated, around testes disappears very slowly on under-feeding. Fat accumulated around testes, disturbs thermoregulatory mechanism and hence there is poor semen quality. Protein deficiencies normally do not occur. Deficiencies of protein, as low as less than 2% in ration would cause loss of libido and less semen production. Vit. A is necessary for normal spermatogenesis. 35-100 µg of Vit. A/kg body weight/day is sufficient for normal reproduction and this requirement is met normally easily. Deficiencies of other vitamins have not been recorded in domestic male animals. Deficiencies of iron, copper and cobalt cause anemia, loss of appetite, loss of weight and mild adverse influence on reproduction in male animals. Deficiencies of calcium, manganese, zinc, potassium and iodine have not been proved to be associated with infertility in male animals.

Chapter 11

Storage and Transportation of Semen

STORAGE

Some common precautions in the storage of diluted semen are :
1. Protection from cold shock,
2. Protection from contamination by water, urine and chemicals,
3. Protection from excessive jerks and agitation,
4. Protection from exposure to air and
5. Protection from exposure to direct sunlight.

Vigorous shaking of semen in the presence of air leads to oxidation of cytochronome enzyme within spermatozoa.

Storage of semen at room temperature(ambient temperature)

The semen at ambient temperature should be stored in 1ml ampoules or vials i.e. each ampoule/vial should contain only one insemination dose. The ampoules/vials should be completely filled with semen and as little air space as possible should be left in ampoule/vial. The ampoules/vials should be wrapped in cotton and then put in paper bag. Exposure to light should be avoided. The semen packets may be put in wooden boxes for transportation.

Storage of semen at refrigeration temperature (5°C)

The glassware containing semen should be well cleaned and sterilized. The tube containing extended semen should be put in a beaker or jar containing clean water at room temperature and both should be kept at the bottom (not top) of the refrigerator to cool slowly. The semen tube should be properly covered with aluminum foil or screw cap. During use, the extended semen should be taken out for minimum possible period and should always be protected from thermal shock, agitation and exposure to light.

Storage of deep freezed semen in liquid nitrogen

The frozen semen is stored always dipped in liquid nitrogen. It is also necessary that liquid nitrogen container should not be damaged. The room of storing liquid nitrogen containers (containing frozen semen) should be properly ventilated and cool. The liquid nitrogen containers should always remain loaded with cap except during taking out or putting in frozen semen or during pouring of liquid nitrogen. The number as well as length of exposure of frozen semen outside liquid nitrogen should be kept as minimum as possible. The level of the liquid nitrogen should be regularly checked.

TRANSPORTATION

The role of artificial insemination would be much more if the extended semen from genetically superior sires is widely distributed at distant places and in wide spread areas.

The **semen in ambient temperature dilutors** is generally packed in 1 ml dose (single inseminating dose). The vials should be wrapped in cotton and then put in a paper bag. Such paper bag may be put in wooden box having inner layer made up of thermocol. In this container the semen may be dispatched to places of need. The containers may be labeled as :

- Living biological product.
- Rush it.

The tube containing **chilled diluted semen** may be transported through cycle, motorcycle, bus or train. Whatever may be the mode of transportation, it should always be kept in mind that :

1. Moisture should not enter the tube.
2. Semen tube/vial should be prevented from breaking.
3. Jerks should be minimized to their maximum.
4. The semen tube should not come in close contact with ice.

The transportation of the chilled liquid semen may be done either in thermos flask or in insulated cartons. In thermos, there should be a layer of crushed ice at the bottom and then a good layer of cotton/wool. Then the tube containing chilled semen may be put. It should be noted that refrigeration temperature dilutors work well at 4 to 5°C. The ice (0°C temperature) would kill sperms in refrigeration temperature dilutors. Hence it is necessary to ensure that the semen tube does not come in direct contact with ice. Also the semen tubes should be water tight. For shipping chilled liquid semen in cartons, the water tight semen tubes are wrapped in paper and are put in double insulating bag (may be rubber bag). The arrangement is such that moisture is absorbed by the paper, breaking of semen tube is prevented and too close contact of semen with ice is avoided. Both, the semen tube in insulated cover and ice bag in insulated cover are put in cartons. The semen tubes are kept in cartons in straight upright position. The shipping carton is labeled as :

- Living biological product.
- Handle with care.
- ↑ This side up.
- Rush it.

The **frozen semen** is transported dipped in liquid nitrogen. The main precautions in the transportation of frozen semen are :

1. It should be ensured that the level of liquid nitrogen does not go down and the semen straws/ampoules remain dipped in liquid nitrogen.

2. Liquid nitrogen containers should also be protected from damage during transportation. For safety, liquid nitrogen containers may be put in tin boxes having hole at top. This would also protect the vacuum seal of the liquid nitrogen container. The use of rubber bottom pads and rubber belts greatly aid in preventing damage to the liquid nitrogen containers.

3. Frictional damages to the liquid nitrogen containers should be avoided. Liquid nitrogen containers should either be lifted by attendants or trolley with wheels should be used. Liquid nitrogen containers should not be slipped against the ground with friction.

4. Undesired material should not be put in the liquid nitrogen containers.

5. Transportation with public vehicle should be avoided. It may lead to serious consequences.

6. The consignee should be well informed about details of semen, date of dispatch and mode of transportation etc.

7. The container should be labeled as :

   • Living biological product.

   • Handle with care.

   • Rush it.

   • ↑ This side up.

Chapter 12

Biochemistry and Metabolism of Semen

BIOCHEMISTRY

The semen ejaculated is a mixture of spermatozoa and the secretions from testes, epididymis, ampullary glands, vesicular glands, prostate gland and bulbourethral glands (Fig. 12.1).

Sperm cells constitute on an average about 10% of the semen by volume in bull and 2-5% of the semen by volume in boar. On an average the contribution of secretion from vesicular glands in 32-38%, the contribution from epididymis is 31-36% and the contribution from both the prostate and the bulbourethral glands is 31-32%. The water content in the semen ranges from 85 to 98%. During natural service, seminal plasma serves as vehicle for spermatozoa transport as well as it protects spermatozoa from damage.

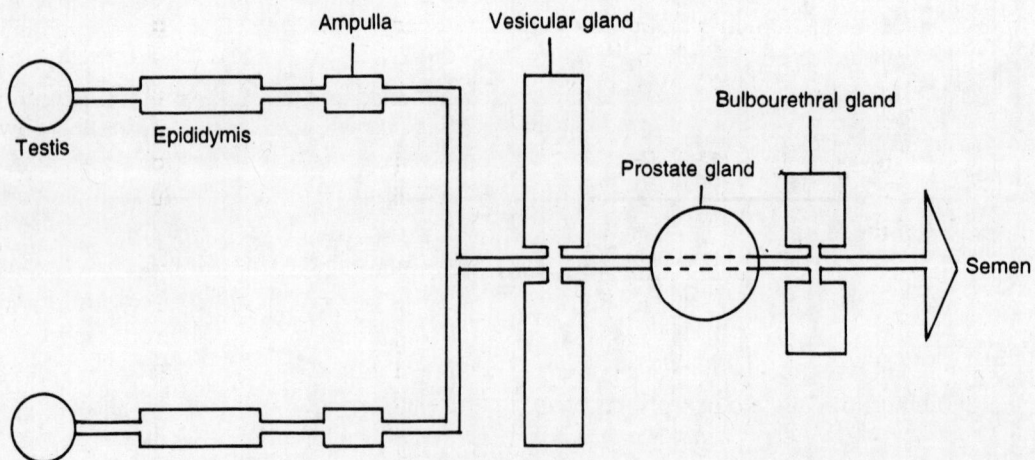

Fig. 12.1. Schematic diagram to show that ejaculated semen is composed of testicular fluid together with contributions from epididymis, ampulla, vesicular gland, prostate gland and bulbourethral gland.

The semen contains a wide variety of organic and inorganic substances like amino acids, peptides, proteins, lipids, sugars (fructose, sorbitol, mannose), ergothioneine, glycerylphosphoryl-choline, ascorbic acid, citric acid, fatty acid, numerous enzymes, seminal plasmin (antimicrobial constituent), immunoglobulins (mainly IgA class), several hormones (androgens, estrogens, prosta-glandins, FSH, LH, Chorionic gonadotropin like substances, growth hormone, insulin, glucagon, prolactin, relaxin and thyroid releasing hormones etc.), vitamins and inorganic ions including heavy metals.

The value of different substances vary in between species, within species, in between different individuals, in different samples of the same animal and in different fractions of the single ejaculate eg. presperm fraction of stallion's ejaculate has low concentration of citric acid and ergothioneine, sperm rich fraction is rich in ergothioneine and post sperm fraction is rich in citric acid.

The **pH** of the freshly collected semen on an average is 6.8 in bull, 7.4 in stallion, 6.8 in ram, 7.4 in boar and 6.7 in dog. As the live spermatozoa metabolize the organic substances, the pH of the semen drops. In bull the pH of the freshly collected semen at 37°C drops about 0.32 in one hour. Greater is the concentration of spermatozoa in the semen sample, greater is the drop in pH. Similarly the pH of semen would drop faster with greater motility of the spermatozoa. Lactic acid is formed on storage of semen and pH is lowered down. This lowering of pH is detrimental to spermatozoa. pH does not influence the oxygen utilization but rather it influences fructolysis. There is higher fructolysis at higher pH.

Fructose is the normal **sugar** providing energy to spermatozoa in ruminants (bull, ram and goat). It is low in boar, very low in stallion and is absent in dog (seminal vesicles are absent in dog and cat). Fructose is mainly produced in the seminal vesicles and is derived from glucose. The average levels of fructose (mg/100 ml) are 500 in bull, 250 in sheep and goat, 10 in boar and 2 in stallion. Spermatozoa can utilized glucose also for energy as well. Sorbitol is a sugar alcohol and can be oxidized to fructose and provides a source of energy. Mannose can also be utilized as a source of energy. Inositol (from seminal vesicles) occurs in high concentration in boar semen and acts chiefly as osmotic pressure regulator. **Ergothioneine** (a sulphydryl containing compound) is secreted from vesicular glands and occurs in appreciable amount in boar and stallion semen. Ergothioneine is also uniquely present in stallion's ampullary glands. **Glyceryl-phosphorylcholine** is a distinctive component of the epididymal secretion.

The sticky, gelatinous, get like material from the bulbourethral glands make up about 20-30% of the total porcine ejaculate. This gel like substance seals the cervix and prevents back flow of semen during natural service. (This gel fraction is generally discarded in artificial insemination practice). This gel like fraction is also produced substantially in certain individuals or in certain ejaculates in stallions.

The bull semen contains several **inorganic ions** like sodium, potassium, magnesium, calcium, chlorides and phosphates. Heavy metals (eg Cu, Fe, Co, Mn, Zn, Pb, Cd, and Hg) are found in traces. Phosphates are essential for energy metabolism. Sulphates, tartarates, citrates and phosphates are favourable and prevent swelling of the spermatozoa. Chlorides, iodides, chlorates, nitrates and thiocyantes are harmful and aid in swelling of spermatozoa. Potassium ions are chiefly cellular and are important in cellular metabolism. Potassium ions are necessary for optimal spermatozoa motility. Sodium ions are in more amount compared to potassium ions and are in abundance in seminal plasma. The concentration of calcium ions is less compared to either sodium or potassium. Calcium ions depress motility, respiration and glycolysis and are generally not added in semen extenders. The concentration of magnesium ions in the semen is very little. Magnesium ions have important role in metabolism. For potassium ions to improve glycolysis and motility, the presence of magnesium ions is necessary. Heavy metals (Cu, Fe, Co, Mn, Pb, Zn, Cd and Hg) are in general toxic to spermatozoa. Fe and Cu are generally consistently spermicidal because of their binding with sulphahydryl (SH) group. Glutathion and glycine are beneficial in such toxicity due to their chelating nature with heavy metals. Semen characteristics of domestic animals are given in Table 12.1.

Table 12.1. Semen characteristics of domestic animals

Characteristic	Bull	Stallion	Ram	Boar	Dog
pH	6.8	7.4	6.8	7.4	6.7
Range of pH	6.4 - 7.8	7.2 - 7.8	6.0 - 7.3	7.3 - 7.8	6.0 - 6.8
Fructose (mg/100 ml)	500	2	250	10	—
Sorbitol (mg/100 ml)	10-140	40	100	12	—
Inositol (mg/100 ml)	35	30	12	500	—
Ergothioneine (mg/100 ml)	0	40-110	0	17	—
Glyceryl phosphorylcholine (GPC) (mg/100 ml)	350	40-100	1650	110-240	180
Citric acid (mg/100 ml)	700	25	150	175	Traces
Protine (gm/100 ml)	6.8	1.0	5.0	3.7	—
Sodium (mg/100 ml)	230	100-250	180	600	90
Potassium (mg/100 ml)	150	70-100	90	200	—
Calcium (mg/100 ml)	40	26	6	6	—
Magnesium (mg/100 ml)	8	9	6	10	—
Chloride (mg/100 ml)	200	450	86	30	—

- Antiagglutinin prevents head to head agglutination of spermatozoa and is found in seminal plasma.
- Dog semen has 7 times more level of copper and 20 times more level of zinc compared to blood.

SPERMATOZOAL METABOLISM

The motility of the spermatozoa though speaks about its physiological status, is not an accurate predictor of its fertilizing capacity. The energy for spermatozoal motility is derived from intra-cellular stores of ATP. The breakdown of ATP is regulated by endogenous level of cyclic AMP (cAMP). cAMP also has direct effect on sperm motility. The spermatozoa possess the enzymes necessary for biochemical metabolism i.e. glycolysis (Embden-Meyerhof pathway), tricarboxylic acid cycle, fatty acid oxidation, electron transport and hexose monophosphate shunt.

Anaerobic metabolism (glycolysis or fructolysis) (Fig. 12.2)

Anaerobic metabolism is the predominant metabolism occurring in the cytosol. Under anaerobic condition i.e. in the absence of oxygen, spermatozoa can break down glucose, fructose (mainly) or mannose to lactic acid. Fructose is present in most of the mammalian semen. Fructose is found in seminal vesicles and is derived from glucose. In the epididymis, spermatozoa are immotile as they do not have access (approach) to fructose. Lactose (the milk sugar) is not metabolized by the spermatozoa. This is because of this glycolytic activity (or more correctly the fructolytic activity),

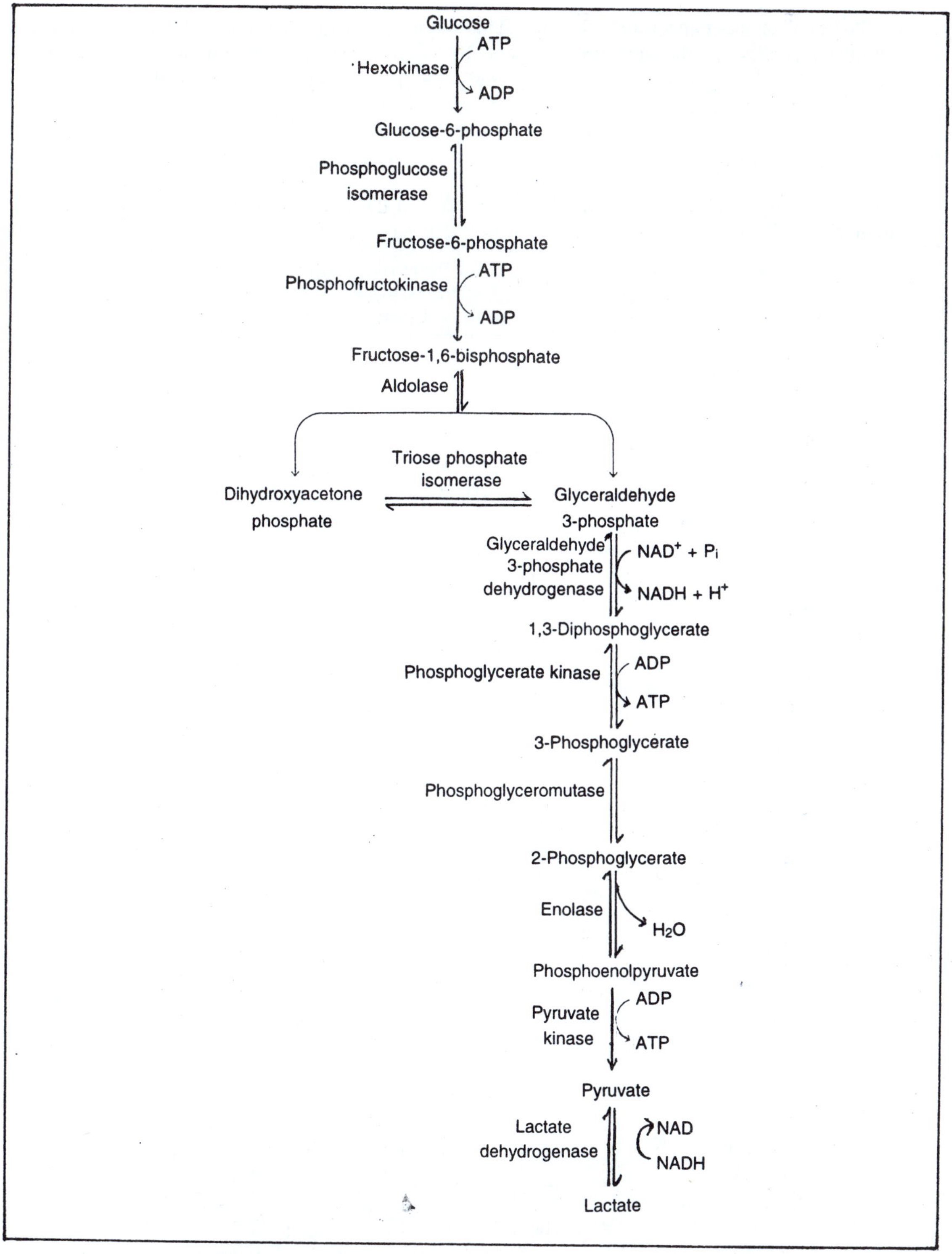

Glucose

ATP

Hexokinase

ADP

Glucose-6-phosphate

Phosphoglucose
isomerase

Fructose-6-phosphate

ATP

Phosphofructokinase

ADP

Fructose-1,6-bisphosphate

Aldolase

Dihydroxyacetone
phosphate

Triose phosphate
isomerase

Glyceraldehyde
3-phosphate

Glyceraldehyde
3-phosphate
dehydrogenase

$NAD^+ + P_i$

$NADH + H^+$

1,3-Diphosphoglycerate

Phosphoglycerate kinase

ADP

ATP

3-Phosphoglycerate

Phosphoglyceromutase

2-Phosphoglycerate

Enolase

H_2O

Phosphoenolpyruvate

Pyruvate
kinase

ADP

ATP

Pyruvate

Lactate
dehydrogenase

NAD

NADH

Lactate

Fig. 12.2. Anaerobic metabolism (glycolysis or fructolysis).

spermatozoa survive under anaerobic condition. This characteristic of anaerobic metabolism (glycolysis or fructolysis) is vital in the storage of semen for use in artificial insemination. The fructose contents as well as fructolysis index of buffalo bull semen is less than in cattle bull semen and this may be the reason for poor keeping quality of buffalo bull semen.

Aerobic metabolism (Fig. 12.3)

Spermatozoa use a variety of substrates in the presence of oxygen. The aerobic metabolism occurs in mitochondria. In the aerobic metabolism, the lactate or pyrutate obtained from fructolysis of

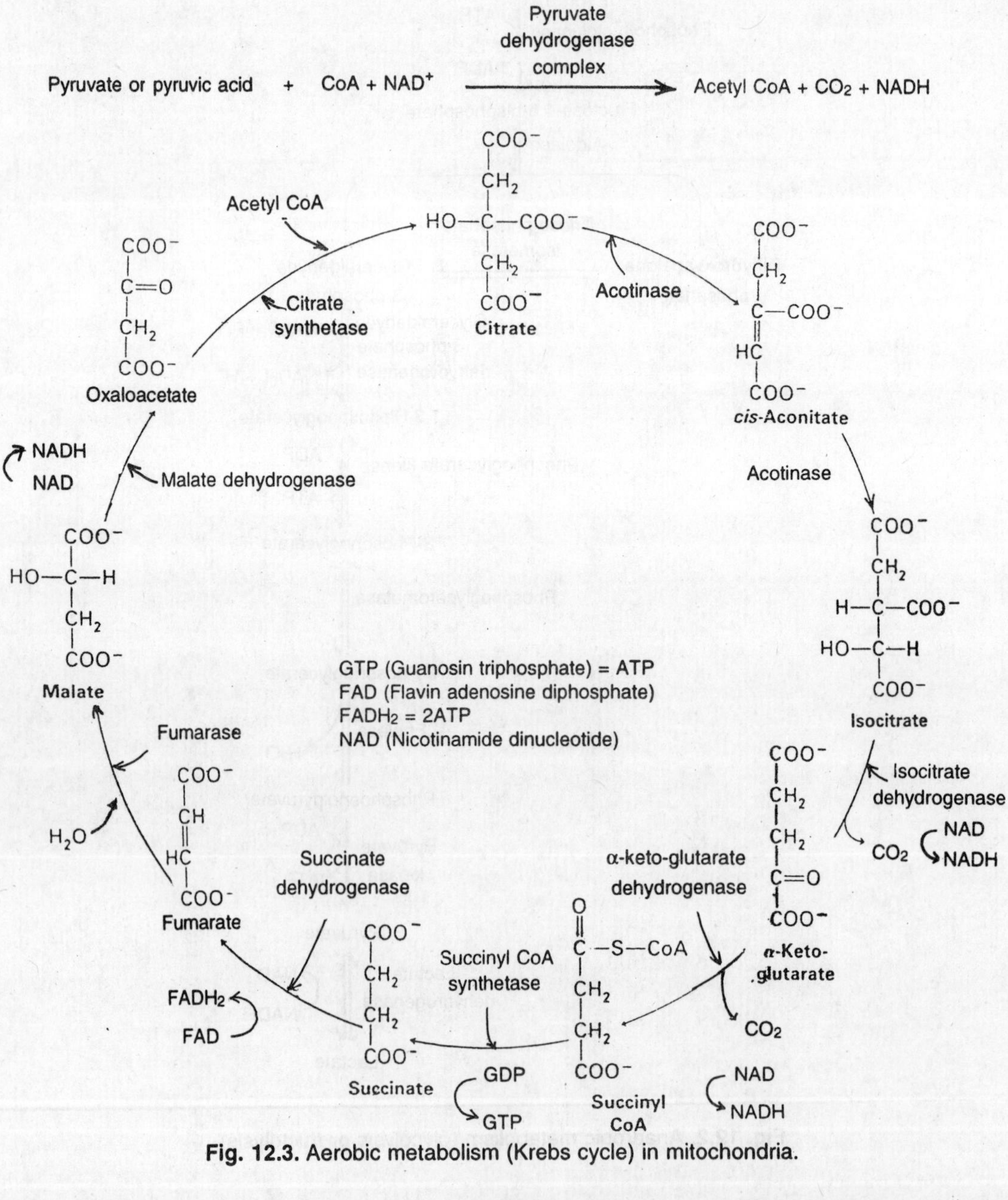
Pyruvate or pyruvic acid + CoA + NAD+
Pyruvate dehydrogenase complex
Acetyl CoA + CO2 + NADH
Acetyl CoA
Citrate synthetase
Citrate
Acotinase
cis-Aconitate
Acotinase
Isocitrate
Isocitrate dehydrogenase
CO2
NAD
NADH
α-keto-glutarate dehydrogenase
α-Keto-glutarate
CO2
NAD
NADH
Succinyl CoA
Succinyl CoA synthetase
GDP
GTP
Succinate
Succinate dehydrogenase
FADH2
FAD
Fumarate
Fumarase
H2O
Malate
Malate dehydrogenase
NADH
NAD
Oxaloacetate
GTP (Guanosin triphosphate) = ATP
FAD (Flavin adenosine diphosphate)
FADH2 = 2ATP
NAD (Nicotinamide dinucleotide)

Fig. 12.3. Aerobic metabolism (Krebs cycle) in mitochondria.

sugars (anaerobic metabolism) are utilized to yield carbon dioxide and water. The aerobic metabolism is considerably more efficient in the production of energy compard to fructolysis.

Using anaerobic and aerobic pathways, the spermatozoa convert most of the energy in to ATP. Most of the ATP is used for spermatozoa motility, some is used in the active transport process of spermatozoa membrane. These active transport processes prevent loss of vital ions from sperm cell.

Chapter 13

The Examination of the Bull for Breeding Soundness

The bulls are examined for the adequacy of reproductive functions. It must be borne in mind that in addition to the proper functioning of the genital organs there should be perfect neuromusculoskeletal and hooves system for proper coitus and ejaculation. The examination of the bull for breeding soundness though is rarely required (compared to females) but needs clinical competency, acquaintance with bull's psychology, patience, common sense, knowledge of clinical pathology and sometimes also the sensefull courage and athletic power in the veterinarian. Further, the examination of the bull should be conducted very carefully and thoroughly in a preplanned and systematic procedure so that no system/part of significance is left unexamined. All bulls must be considered extremely dangerous. Bulls should never be trusted, howsoever they had been gentle in the past. The bulls should be properly restrained before examination. Nose rings are of utmost importance in restraining the bulls. The bulls should be well secured in a tie stall. It is better to make slow approach to the bull, talking in tones of kindness. The first approach should be towards shoulder area rather than to the back of the bull. The sensations to the bull should be pleasurable. During examination sudden moves, loud noise, sudden entry of strange persons etc. should be avoided so that the bull is not excited. The name/number of the bull together with permanent identification marks on its body should be well recorded for each bull. Each finding should be recorded. The basic steps for evaluation of the breeding soundness in males include :

1. History (anamnesis)
2. General physical examination
3. Special clinical examination of the reproductive system
    (a) Examination of externalia
    (b) Examination of internalia
4. Semen examination
5. Other diagnostic tests i.e. Campylobacteriosis, Trichomoniasis, Brucellosis, Leptospirosis, Tuberculosis, Johne's disease, Q. fever, Anaplasmosis, IBR-IPV infection etc.

HISTORY

In order to assess the genetic potential of the bull, the history regarding the Dam's yield, Grand Dam's yield and whenever possible, the yield of the progeny should be noted. It is now becoming necessary in India that the genetic group of the bull and the percentage of the exotic blood in the bull be recorded so as to select bull of desired genetic group with desired exotic blood percentage as per need. The fertility records of the bull should be noted. The records of the females bred by the bull in question should also be critically analysed for the incidence of abnormal discharge, abortion, and delayed return of estrum following service. History regarding operations for hernia, penile deviation etc should be collected, as such defects are not desirable and may be transmitted to the progeny. The records of all possible vaccinations should be collected. The examiner should also determine the presence of recessive genes in the bull which by mating with females having similar genes would be carried to the off-springs and prove lethal, semi lethal or would be undesirable.

GENERAL PHYSICAL EXAMINATION

The animals cannot communicate any information verbally regarding their diseases. The examination of the bull should be conducted in such a way that no organ/part of the body is omitted without investigation. It is always better that the examination is conducted in a preplanned manner. The general physical examination would include :

1. Physical condition
2. Integument and body wall
3. Digestive system
4. Urinary system
5. Circulatory system
6. Lymphatic system
7. Respiratory system
8. Locomotor (neuromusculoskeletal and hooves, NMSH) system

Physical condition

The physical condition is assessed by simple inspection. The bull may be normal, obese, thin or emaciated. The overall condition should be satisfactory. Bulls should be neither too fat nor too thin. The bulls should be alert and should respond to external stimuli, such as movement and sound. Abnormal behavior, if any, should be considered of clinical significance wanting further investigations. Unusual behavior may be due to pain. The vices, if any, should be noted. Behavior of the bull during eating, defecation and urination should be noted carefully. The vision of the bull should be normal. The anterior portion of the bull near the shoulder region should be massive and well developed. The hump in zebu bulls should be massive, well developed and erect. Hump leaning on one side, though have no significance as far the breeding soundness is concerned, but such bulls are generally not preferred by the breeders. The bulls should have masculine voice and should have some aggressive and masculine nature and should not be docile and of feminine nature. The skin coat should appear smooth and shiny.

Integument and body wall

There should not be inguinal, umbilical or other hernias. Even surgically repaired hernias may not be recommended for the selection of bulls. During mounting, ejaculation and during thrust, the muscles are stretched and the condition may further deteriorate each time.

Digestive system

The variations in the bull's appetite should be assessed and whenever the appetite is impaired, the cause should be investigated. Disturbances in eating, drinking, prehension, mastication of food and deglutition (swallowing) should be noted carefully. The mucus membrane of the oral cavity, tongue and teeth should be examined. The bull should have enough teeth to allow them to eat. Bulls with defective teeth (e.g. lesions) or less number of teeth would rapidly lose weight. It would be better if fecal samples are examined for the presence of intestinal parasites etc., so that the severely affected bulls are left out.

Urinary system

The urinary system should be given full attention. The important aspects which need attention include, the posture during urination, the frequency of urination, the evidence of pain during urination and the changes in the quality and quantity of the urine.

Circulatory system

Generally the cardiovascular diseases are less commonly diagnosed in bovines. Attention should be paid to diagnose cardiovascular disorders in the selection of bulls. Heart beats should be recorded. The diseases like dilatation of heart, traumatic pericarditis, myocarditis etc. should be diagnosed. Bulls with poor exercise tolerance and difficult breathing should be thoroughly investigated.

Lymphatic system

The lymph nodes are examined by visual inspection and palpation. The size, pain reaction, lobulation, consistency, temperature of overlying skin and abscess formation etc. should be noted in lymph glands. In selected cases, biopsy specimens may be obtained for histopathological examination. The iliac, mesenteric and deep inguinal lymph nodes may be easily examined during the palpation of internalia.

Respiratory system

The respiratory system should be assessed by noting movements of ribs, sternum and the flank, preferably in standing animal. The rate of respiration, type of respiration, rhythm (regularity) of respiration and depth of respiration should be noted. Painful respiration may occur in pleurisy and peritonitis. Abdominal type of respiration may occur in pleurisy or due to pain in thoracic wall. Any unusual symptom such as coughing and nasal discharge should be thoroughly investigated.

Locomotor (neuromusculoskeletal and hooves, NMSH) system

Together with the male genital organs including penis, testes, accessory sex glands and other supporting structures, the neuromusculoskeletal and hooves system (NMSH) make a very important part of semen delivery system. It may be noted that during coitus and ejaculation, the bull is engaged in highly coordinated movements and during this period the total weight of the bull (Approx. 450-500 kg) is supported by hind limbs only. Further, while bearing the weight, the hind limbs are brought in nearly full extension during the act of forceful thrust leading to ejaculation. Hence, it is extremely important that due emphasis should be given on conformation, particularly of the hind limbs and the neuromusculoskeletal and hooves system. The joints, their angles, base of the foot, symmetry of hooves, weight bearing capacity and gait of the bull should be thoroughly examined. The conformation of the rear legs should be observed from the side as well as from the rear. The medial and lateral hooves should be symmetrical and in close apposition to each other. The gait should be normal and well coordinated. Hind limbs should have weight bearing capacity. There should be no arthritis, no pain and no indication of any paralysis. The asthesia (feeling sensitivity) of the limbs should be normal.

Rear legs conformation as seen from side

Normal conformation

In normal bull the angles of the tarsal joints should be proper and should be neither excessively small nor excessively large. Also the metatarsophalangeal joints should be proper and should be neither curved and weak nor too straight (Fig. 13.1).

Abnormal conformations

(a) **Sickle hock conformation :** The angle of the tarsus is small. This condition may lead to swelling in the hock joint and lameness (Fig. 13.2).

(b) **Postiness/Post-Legged Bulls :** The angle of the tarsus is large. The bulls having this defect lack proper angulation of the stifle and hock joints. The angle of the metatarsophalangeal joint is reduced. In such bulls the pastern is noticeably weakened. The condition is often bilateral in bulls and is evident by 1-3 years of age. In post legged bulls the peroneus tertius and gastrocnemius muscles (these two muscles cause the stifle and hock joints to flex or extend together) are so structured anatomically that the joints (stifle and hock) remain continuously extended (Fig. 13.3). In such bull cruciate ligament and meniscus may be suppressed. Primary postiness is a conformational defect and generally there is no pain in early primary postiness. Secondary postiness may also develop in older bulls, either unilaterally or bilaterally. Secondary postiness is generally a pain-sparling action.

(c) **Camped behind :** In such bulls the angle of the tarsus is extremely large. The rear foot is stayed far behind. The affected bulls shift their rear legs frequently in order to find a position of comfort. Such bulls usually swayback (Fig. 13.4).

Rear legs conformation as seen from back

Normal conformation

In normal bull the axes of the stifle, tarsal and fetlock joints approximately intersect the rear limb in right and left sagittal planes (Fig. 13.5).

Abnormal conformations

(a) **Bow legged or Narrow base or Medial rotation :** In this defect the hind limbs are curved medially and as a result the outside wall of the hoof is compressed. The out side toe may be curled. Such bulls show lameness of varying degree. Such bulls require frequent trimming of hooves (Fig. 13.6).

(b) **Cow-hocked or Wide base or Lateral rotation or Toed-out stance :** In this defect the hind limbs are curved laterally (Fig. 13.7). This fault is usually seen associated with sickle-hock conformation. In this defect the inside hoof is compressed and the bull may show lameness of varying degree.

Other defects

(a) **Progressive posterior paresis :** The incidence is high in older bulls and the disease is rarely seen in younger bulls, below 6 years of age. The skin asthesia (feeling sensitivity) usually remains

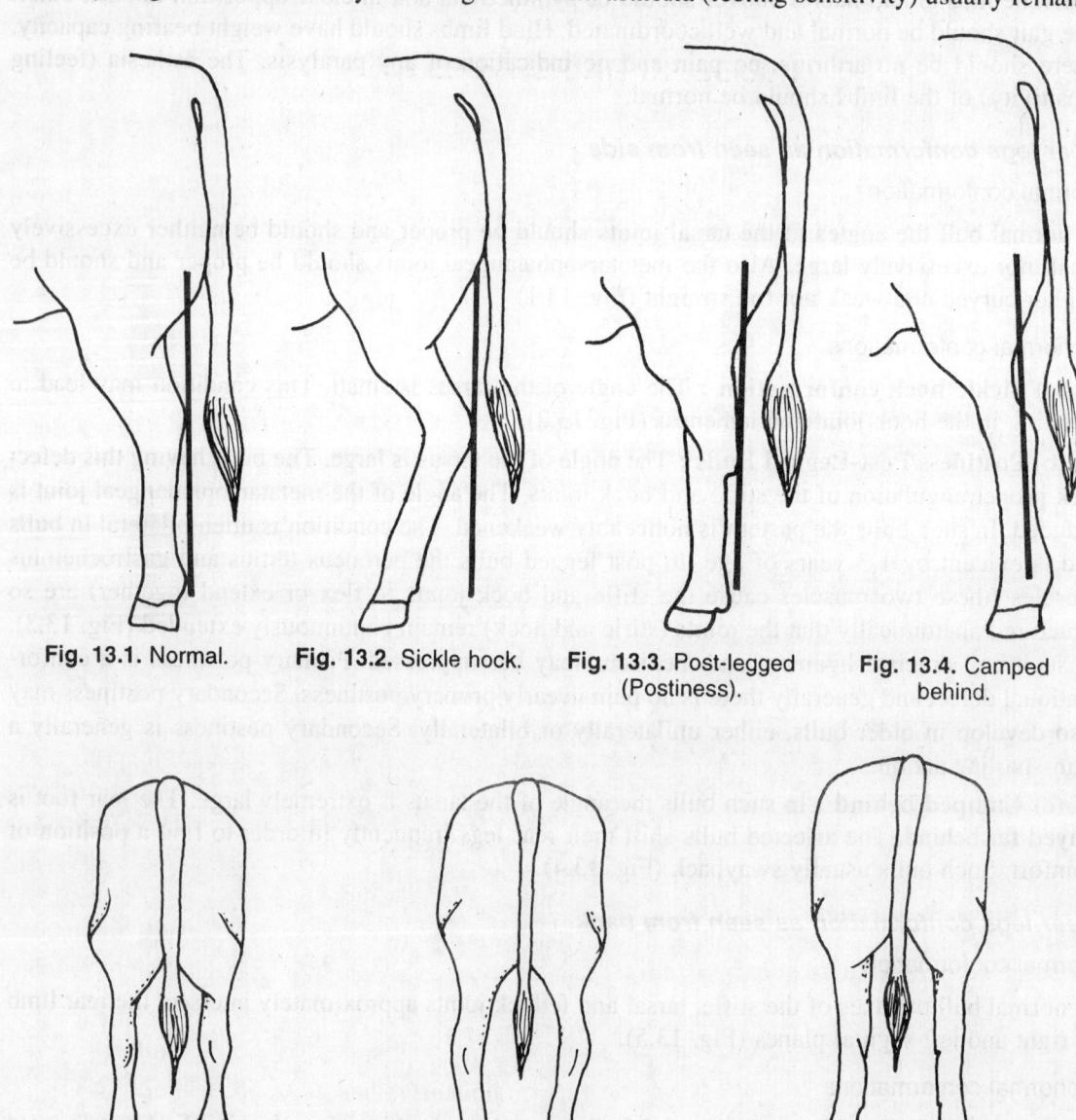

Fig. 13.1. Normal.   **Fig. 13.2.** Sickle hock.   **Fig. 13.3.** Post-legged (Postiness).   **Fig. 13.4.** Camped behind.

Fig. 13.5. Normal.   **Fig. 13.6.** Bow-legged or Narrow base or Medial rotation.   **Fig. 13.7.** Cow-hocked or Wide base or Lateral rotation or Toed-out stance.

intact but there is slow onset of ataxia (inability to coordinate voluntary movements). There is impairment exclusively on motor function because of destruction of motor nerve fibers or neurons in the spinal cord. The condition worsens with the time. The terminal part of rectum and anus may also be paralyzed and hence defecation may involve abdominal press. The urinary bladder may not contract and urination may occur as spillover.

(b) **Crampiness or Spastic syndrome or Stretches or Neuromuscular spasticity :** The disease occurs only in mature bulls. There are cramps (Cramp= involuntary and painful contractions of voluntary muscles) bilaterally when the bull is in the standing position or when the bull is rising. Such signs are not noted during recumbency. The disease involves highly complex postural reflex system.

(c) **Spastic paresis (Elso heel) :** The disease occurs in young bull (generally below 1 year of age) The disease is usually unilateral. There are chronic contractions of gastrocnemius and superficial digital flexor muscles and the result is that the hock and stifle joints are maintained in nearly full extension. Trembling muscle contractions are seen in the affected limb, particularly when the bull is rising. The affected limb usually swing in pendulous way, points anteriolaterally, may not touch the ground and hence appears short.

SPECIAL CLINICAL EXAMINATION OF THE REPRODUCTIVE ORGANS

Examination of the externalia

The scrotum with testes, the penis and prepuce make the externalia. The externalia should be examined carefully after the animal is properly restrained so that the examiner is well protected from injuries. The testes, scrotum, epididymis, penis and prepuce should be examined using both hands. The testes should be examined visually and by palpation for their size, shape, consistency, position and adhesions with the scrotum. In case the size of the two testes differs, there should be further careful investigation. The semen production is closely related to testicular size and consistency. The scrotum should be free from fat and varicoceles(an enlargement of the veins of the spermatic cord or those of the scrotum). The abaxial surface should be convex. The scrotal wall should be thin and flexible. The measurements of scrotal circumstance are accurate predictors of sperm out put. The head, body and tail of the epididydmis should be examined carefully by palpation for detecting abscesses or unusual enlargement. Normally the body of the epididymis lies caudo-medially and the head of the epididymis lies anteriolaterally on testicular surface.

Any unusual softness, firmness, atrophy, hypertrophy, swelling and pain etc. should be carefully investigated. Small testes, testes held close to the body wall hypoplasia—both unilateral and bilateral, cryptorchidism and scrotal hernia lead to poor prognosis. Testicular shape, measurements and consistency in bull are given in Table 13.1.

Table 13.1. Testicular shape, measurements and consistency in bull

Shape (testis)	Oval
Length (testis)	10.0-15.0 cm
Diameter (testis)	5.0-8.5 cm
Weight (testis)	200.0-500.0 gm
Scrotal circumference	32.0-36.0 cm
Consistency	Turgescent yet resilient

The penis and the prepuce can be examined at the time of semen collection using artificial vagina and can also be examined by palpation. There should be full penile development. There should not be any inflammation, penile fracture, anatomical abnormality and adhesions etc. The preputial cavity should be examined for adhesions, pathological lesions pathological discharge, trauma and anatomical abnormalities e.g. presence of penile frenulum (Fig. 13.8). Eversion of the prepuce is commonly seen in zebu bulls and such bulls are more prone to preputial damage (Fig. 13.9). A very pendulous prepuce most often seen in zebu bulls predisposes the bull to preputial lesions (Fig. 13.10) because the exposed preputial membrane may get easily infected.

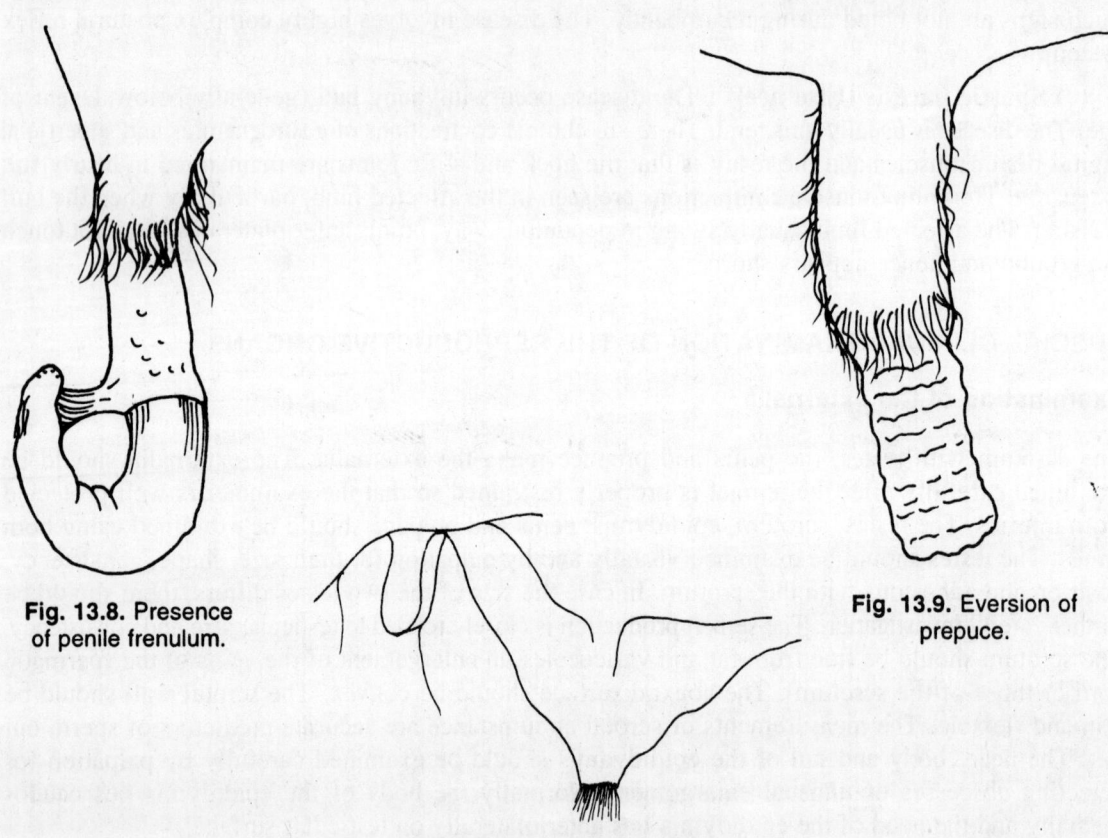

Fig. 13.8. Presence of penile frenulum.

Fig. 13.9. Eversion of prepuce.

Fig. 13.10. Pendulous sheath.

Examination of the internalia (Fig. 13.11)

The pelvic and abdominal genital organs constitute the internalia. For the proper examination of the accessory sex glands, the rectal examination of the bull is essential.

The ampullae

The ampulla is the enlarged terminal glandular portion of the vas deferens. In bull the normal length is 10-12 cm and the diameter is 1.0-1.5 cm. The ampullae can be palpated as broadened terminal parts of vas deferens lying dorsal to the neck of the bladder, pass caudally under the prostate body and open in pelvic urethra through a rounded prominence called as "colliculus seminalis". The ampullae can be readily palpated. Hypoplasia or aplasia of the ampullae is rarely

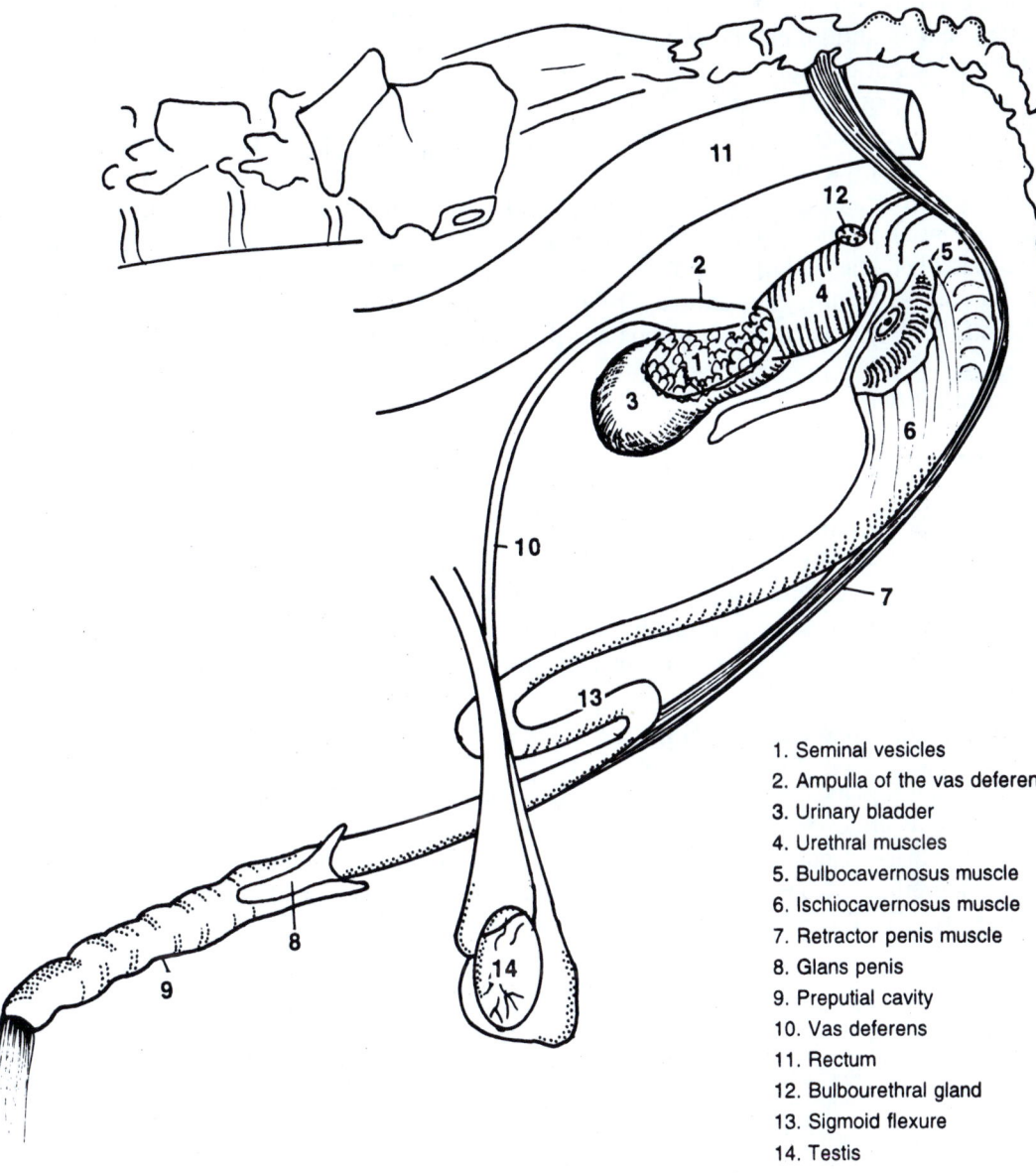

1. Seminal vesicles
2. Ampulla of the vas deferens
3. Urinary bladder
4. Urethral muscles
5. Bulbocavernosus muscle
6. Ischiocavernosus muscle
7. Retractor penis muscle
8. Glans penis
9. Preputial cavity
10. Vas deferens
11. Rectum
12. Bulbourethral gland
13. Sigmoid flexure
14. Testis

Fig. 13.11. Reproductive organs of the bull.

noticed. Ampullitis is not recognized easily. However, higher incidence of infection is noticed at necropsy. These glands are absent in dog.

The vesicular glands

The vesicular glands are located on pelvic floor on each side of the ampullae. The secretion of these glands add volume, nutrition and buffers in the semen. The glands open in pelvic urethra near the opening of ampullae. The normal vesicular gland is about 10-15 cm long and 2-4 cm in diameter. The glands are elongated and have distinct lobulations. The normal consistency of the vesicular gland is soft in young bulls and becomes firmer (meaty) with age. Normally the gland is flexible but in inflammatory conditions the flexibility may be lost in varying degrees. The seminal vesicles of the buffalo bulls are comparatively smaller and less lobulated. It is generally observed that if one testis is affected, then the seminal vesicle of the same side is also involved. The seminal vesicles are more prone to diseased conditions as compared to other accessory glands. There may be aplasia, hypoplasia, cystic condition and infectious conditions. In acute seminal vesiculitis, there is localized pelvic peritonitis and the gland is enlarged and firm. The semen ejaculates contain purulent exudate. The chronic seminal vesiculitis may not follow the acute phase and the gland becomes enlarged and fibrosed with loss of lobulations. Pain on palpation is usually absent in chronic seminal vesiculitis. The purulent exudate may be present in the semen either consistently or at intervals. These glands are absent in dog and cat.

The prostate gland

The prostate gland is palpated as a thick transverse fibrous band of tissue around the cranial end of pelvic urethra. The gland opens by many ducts in pelvic urethra lateral to "colliculus seminalis" (prominence for the opening of ampullae). The prostate gland has two parts, the body and the pars disseminata. The body is palpable and is 2.5-4.0 cm wide and 1.0-1.5 cm. thick. The pars disseminata surrounds the pelvic urethra and is non-palpable. Dorsally, the pars disseminata is 10-12 cm long and 1.0-1.5 cm thick and is covered by urethral muscles. The gland in bulls is rarely affected (affected commonly in dog). However, inflammatory processes have been detected at necropsy.

The bulbourethral (Cowper's) glands

The bulbourethral glands are paired glands located on either side of pelvic urethra near the ischial arch. The glands are ovoid in shape and have nearly 2-4 cm diameter in bulls. The glands cannot be palpated as these glands are embedded under the bulbospongiosus muscle. Inflammatory processes in the bulbourethral glands have been reported at necropsy but not clinically. Average clinical values are given in Table 13.2. These glands are absent in dog.

Table 13.2. Average clinical values

	Cattle bull	Buffalo bull
Rectal temperature	38.6°C (101.6°F)	38.6°C (101.6°F)
Pulse rate	40-60/min	40-60/min
Respiration rate	16-18/min	16-18/min
Rumen movements	7-8/5 min	7-8/5 min
Haemoglobin (gm %)	11.3	12.9
PCV (%)	33.7	44.3
RBC ($\times 10^6$/mm^3)	5.9	6.8
WBC ($\times 10^3$/mm^3)	7.0	6.7
Differential count		
Neutrophils	29	28
Eosinophils	10	3
Basophils	1	0-1
Lymphocytes	51	60
Monocytes	8-9	7-8

SEMEN EXAMINATION

The semen examination is of great diagnostic value in determining the cause, severity and the degree of the pathological conditions of the testes and other genital organs. The quality of semen is also of value in predicting fertility of the male. Semen quality remains almost constant (varies within narrow limits) for different ejaculates over months or even years in bulls. Under adverse influences the semen quality may deteriorate rapidly but the improvement in the semen quality is slow and it may take months for recovery. There are several parameters to evaluate the semen quality. Usually bulls with good semen samples have good fertility and bulls with poor or very poor semen samples are invariably infertile or sterile. A single test is never sufficient to assess the semen quality and the examiner should be acquainted with several tests to evaluate the semen. The semen should be examined within a shortest possible period after ejaculation and the ejaculate must be properly protected and handled until examination. Measurements of spermatozoa in cattle and buffalo bull are given in Table 13.3. The different tests for semen are :

1. Appearance
2. Colour
3. Volume
4. Mass motility
5. Individual motility
6. Hydrogen ion concentration (pH)
7. Concentration or density of spermatozoa
8. Live spermatozoa percentage
9. Sperm abnormalities
10. Other tests e.g. Catalase test, Resistance to cold shock, Millovanov's resistance test (R-test), Methylene blue reduction test, Resazurin reduction test, Fructolysis index and Oxygen utilization test etc.

Table 13.3. Measurements of spermatozoa (μ)

Parts of spermatozoa	Cattle bull		Buffalo bull	
	Length	Width	Length	Width
Head	9.2-9.3	4.3-5.3	7.4-8.4	4.4-5.0
Neck	—	—	—	—
Middle piece	14.0-16.0	0.75	12.5-13.1	0.7
Tail	45	0.5	43.0-46.0	0.5

Appearance

Translucent samples contain few spermatozoa. Uniform and opaque appearance of the ejaculate is indicative of high spermatozoa concentration. Semen with curdy appearance indicate reproductive infections.

Colour

The colour of the bull semen is milky or creamy white. In some bulls the colour of semen may be light yellow owing to the presence of a harmless pigment "Riboflavin" secreted by the accessory glands and it is of no significance. The appearance and colour of the semen have correlation with spermatozoa concentration in the semen samples.

Appearance and colour	Sperm density
Creamy	1.0-1.2 millions/mm^3
Thin milky	0.5-0.6 millions/mm^3
Watery	< 0.3 millions/mm^3

Bull with Orchitis may donate semen of brownish colour because of blood pigment. Dark red or bloody semen is indicative of blood which may come from tubular genital tract. The presence of *Pseudomonas aeroginosa* organisms may change the semen colour from normal to yellowish green especially if the samples are left at room temperature. Clots or flakes in the semen may be due to the pus that may come from tubular tract or accessory glands.

Volume

Under usual breeding conditions(without any stress) the semen volume in bull does not change much. The semen volume is generally less in young and small sized bulls, excessively used bulls, during incomplete ejaculation and in bulls with seminal vesiculitis. Teasing increases the ejaculate volume. If the low ejaculate volume is accompanied by low spermatozoa concentration, the number of the sperm available would also be low and hence would minimize the use of semen. In bulls the average ejaculate volume is 3-5 ml.

Mass motility

The sperm motility at the time of collection is used as a measure to assess the fertilizing capacity of the semen. It indicates both the sperm concentration and their viability. The epididymal spermatozoa gain motility during the course of ejaculation when they come in contact with the secretions of accessory sex glands. All the motile spermatozoa are live but all the immotile spermatozoa are not dead. The first ejaculate after a period of long sexual rest has poor motility as well as high percentage of dead spermatozoa. The mass motility is influenced by season also. In India spring is supposed to be the best season for initial motility followed by summer. In hot and humid climate the semen motility is adversely affected. Care should be taken to protect the semen sample from cold shock that markedly depresses the spermatozoa motility. Excessive heat, contamination with chemicals, uncleaned and dirty glass wares and contamination with dust etc. also reduce the motility. As a result of sperm motility the whole mass of semen is brought under movement and waves/swirls are created which are readily observed under the microscope. For judging mass motility of the spermatozoa, a drop of freshly collected semen is spread uniformly over a clean grease free and dry slide maintained at 30-35°C and is examined under low power of the microscope with facility of electrically heated stage (spermotherm) to maintain the temperature.

The following descriptive quality and numerical scales are assigned to different waves/swirls motion as observed under the microscope.

Findings under microscope	Descriptive value	Numerical scale
1. Extremely rapid waves and eddies. It is difficult to trace the origin and disappearance of the waves. This indicates that nearly 100% of the spermatozoa are motile.	Excellent	5
2. The waves and eddies are comparatively not so rapid. The swirls are observed to move towards the extremities. This indicates that about 90% of the spermatozoa are motile.	Good	4
3. The waves and eddies are slowly moving and are scattered in the field. This indicates that 50-80% of the spermatozoa are progressively motile.	Fair	3
4. The waves and eddies are absent. Movement of spermatozoa is observed. This indicates that nearly 40% of the spermatozoa are in progressive motion. Other sperms may have oscillating or circular movements.	Poor	2
5. No waves and eddies are observed. Only stationary and throbing movements are observed. This indicates that only upto 20% of the spermatozoa may have progressive movements.	Very poor	1
6. Spermatozoa are non-motile.	All dead	0

The mass motility may further be divided as +5.0, +4.5, +4.0, +3.5, +3.0, +2.5, +2.0, +1.5, +1.0 and +0.5 numerical scales. Though conception may occur with semen samples of poor grade, some workers may reject the semen samples having less than +3 motility scale. +3 and above motility rate is considered desirable for optimal fertility.

Individual motility

The estimate of initial mass motility is not a very precise method. Some weakly motile spermatozoa may be exaggerated by surrounding and very active spermatozoa. For this, the individual spermatozoa are observed under the microscope to estimate the total percentage of motile sperm cells in the ejaculate. For the estimation of individual spermatozoa motility, the semen is diluted(about 1 :100 dilution) in normal saline solution or Ringer's solution. One drop of the diluted semen is put on a clean and dry slide and is covered by cover slip. The slide is examined under high power in a microscope having warm stage facility. The following types of motility may be observed in the spermatozoa.

1. Spermatozoa moving very rapidly in the straight forward direction.

2. Spermatozoa moving in forward circular motion because of defects of middle piece and tail.

3. Spermatozoa moving in reverse circling motion.

4. Spermatozoa showing oscillatory movements and jerks without change of place.

The progressively motile sperm cells of bull may cover a distance of 100 to 120 μ in one second. The percentage of the spermatozoa exhibiting progressive movement is determined. The individual motility rating is done as below :

Progressive motility	Descriptive value
1. 80-100%	Excellent
2. 60-80%	Good
3. 40-60%	Fair
4. 20-40%	Poor
5. 0-20%	Very poor

Hydrogen ion concentration (pH)

The pH value of the semen changes depending upon the concentration and the activity of the spermatozoa and hence no better information can be gained by measuring pH of the semen sample. The pH of the semen sample can be measured using narrow range pH paper. The pH of the bull semen is 6.9 (range 6.4 to 7.5). The pH of the semen is generally 7.0 or higher in excessively used bulls, incomplete ejaculates and in pathological conditions of testes, epididymis, ampullae and the seminal vesicles.

Concentration or density of spermatozoa

The spermatozoa concentration in the bull semen may vary from 0.3 to 2.5 millions/mm^3 (average 1.2 millions/mm^3). The ejaculates collected by electro-ejaculation have more volume and less density because of excess fluid secreted by accessory sex glands. A rapid decrease in the spermatozoa concentration following successive ejaculates is indicative of poor spermatozoa reserve. The bull having spermatozoa concentration below 0.1 million/mm^3 are generally infertile/sterile. The concentration of the spermatozoa may be determined by the following methods :

(a) Macroscopic examination using appearance of colour and consistency

(b) Haemocytometer method

(c) Photoelectric colorimeter method

Macroscopic examination

By visual examination, the estimation of the sperm concentration may be done fairly satisfactorily in samples of high sperm density but in low sperm density semen samples, this method may lead to serious errors. The visual characteristics of bull semen corresponding to spermatozoa density are as below :

Visual characteristics	Sperm concentration
Creamy	2.0 millions/mm^3 and above
Light creamy	1.0 million/mm^3
Milky	0.5 million/mm^3
Cloudy-watery	0.1 million/mm^3
Almost clear and watery	< 0.1 million/mm^3

Haemocytometer method

For measuring the concentration (density) of spermatozoa in the semen sample, haemocytometer may be used in a manner similar to that used for making Red Blood Cells count in blood. The **'Neubauer'** slide (Fig. 13.12) of the haemocytometer has two counting chambers. Each RBC chamber (primary square) is divided into 25 (5×5) secondary squares. Each secondary square is further divided into 16 (4×4) tertiary squares (Fig. 13.13). Thus each primary square is divided into 400 (25×16) tertiary squares. These total 400 tertiary squares measures a total area of 1 mm^2. When a drop is placed under the cover slip in a Neubauer blood cell counting chamber, the thickness of the film is 0.1 mm. Thus the total volume of the semen covering 400 tertiary square is 0.1 mm^3. The semen is diluted at the rate of 1 : 200 in RBC pipette in the diluting medium. However for convenience a higher dilution rate (1 : 1000) is generally preferred.

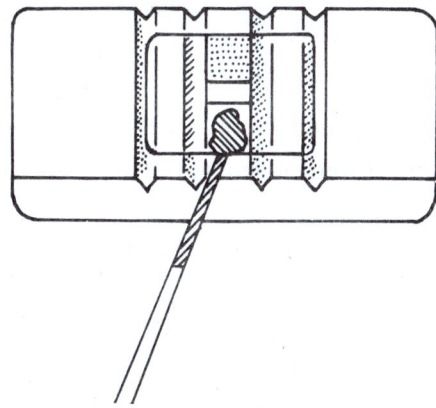

Fig. 13.12. Charging of Neubauer's slide with diluted semen.

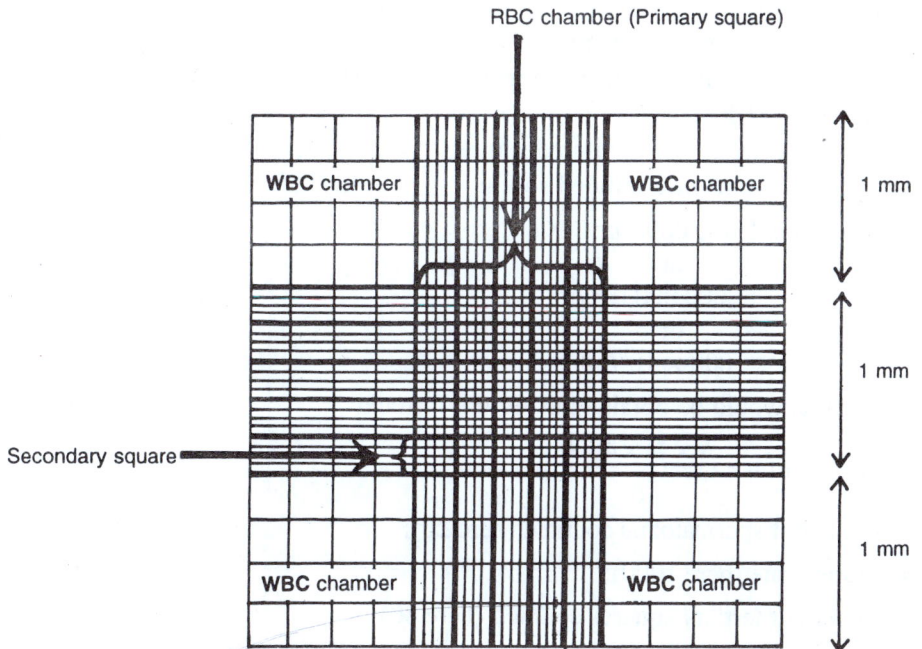

Fig. 13.13. Different squares in Neubauer's slide.

Method

Preparation of Diluting Fluid : Dissolve 0.05 gm of Eosin-y (water soluble) and 1.0 gm of Sodium Chloride in 100 ml distilled water. Eosin may also be dissolved in 100 ml formal saline (1 ml of formalin added to 99 ml of normal saline solution). Formalin kills the spermatozoa and thus the counting is done conveniently.

The diluting fluid of following composition may also be used :

Eosin-y solution (2%)	4 ml
Distilled water	100 ml
Saturated NaCl solution	2 ml

Steps

1. Take 0.1 ml of the well mixed semen.

2. Add to it 9.9 ml of the diluting fluid and mix well (now the dilution is 1 : 100).

3. Take 1 ml of the above diluted semen and add to it 9 ml of diluting fluid (now the dilution is 1 : 1000).

4. Place a drop of diluted semen (1 : 1000 dilution) under the coverslip in a Neubauer blood cell counting chamber. Avoid over flowing. Allow it to settle.

5. Examine under high power objective of the microscope.

6. Count spermatozoa in 80 tertiary squares.

Calculation

Let No. of sperms counted in 80 tertiary squares $= 20$
No. of sperms in 80 tertiary squares $= 20$
No. of sperms in 400 tertiary squares $= 100$
No. of sperms in 0.1 mm^3 of diluted semen $= 100$
Dilution rate is (1 : 1000)
No. of sperms in 0.1 mm^3 of undiluted semen) $= 100,000$
No. of sperms in 1 mm^3 of undiluted serum $= 1,000,000$

So concentration is 1,000,000/mm^3
or
1,000,000,000/ml
or
1000×10^6/ml

The same results would be obtained using the formula

$$\text{Sperm concentration} = \frac{N \times D \times 4000}{n} \text{ per } mm^3$$

where N = Number of spermatozoa counted (here 20);

D = Dilution rate (here 1000);

n = Number of tertiary squares counted (here 80).

$$\text{Sperm concentration} = \frac{N \times D \times 4000}{n} \text{ per } mm^3 = \frac{20 \times 1000 \times 4000}{80} = 1,000,000/mm^3$$

Photoelectric colorimeter method

It is a rapid method for the estimation of sperm concentration in semen samples. The method is based on principle that semen samples with varying spermatozoa concentration absorb varying amount of light. The estimation of spermatozoa concentration using colorimetric method is likely to be erroneous when the semen samples have epithelial cells and other particles in higher concentration.

Various dilutions of the semen are prepared in 3% Sodium citrate dihydrate solution and the number of spermatozoa are standardized in varying dilutions with the help of haemocytometer.

Method

1. Check the instrument.
2. Use preferably red filter (light wavelength of 625 nm).
3. Adjust zero using blank solution (3% Sod. citrate dihydrate solution).
4. Take readings using 0.1 ml of semen of various dilutions (of which the sperm concentration has been assessed with haemocytometer) and 9.9 ml of 3% Sod. citrate dihydrate solution.
5. Plot a graph between photoelectric colorimeter readings and the spermatozoa concentrations. With the help of the graph so prepared, further samples are very easily and rapidly estimated for the concentrations of the spermatozoa.
6. For unknown sample 0.1 ml of semen is added to 9.9 ml of 3% Sod. citrate dihydrate solution and reading of the colorimeter is recorded after adjusting zero with blank solution.
7. Record concentrations with the help of the graph already prepared.

Live spermatozoa

Vital differential staining technique is used for counting live and dead spermatozoa in the semen smears. The Eosin-Nigrosin stain is prepared as below :

Eosin-y (water soluble)	1.67 gm
Nigrosin (water soluble)	10.00 gm
Glass dist. water	100 ml

Eosin stains the dead spermatozoa as pink or red. The live spermatozoa which are alive at the time of staining remain colourless. Live spermatozoa are impermeable to the Eosin stain. Nigrosin provides a blue-black background.

Method

1. Put 5-6 drops of Eosin-Nigrosin stain on a clean slide.
2. Add a drop of semen to the stain and mix gently with the help of a glass rod or platinum loop.
3. After a rest of about 1 min. draw a smear on a clean, grease free slide.
4. Dry in air and examine under microscope.

Sperm abnormalities

The recognition of defective spermatozoa in stained smears provides useful information. The bull's fertility depends upon morphologically normal spermatozoa present in the ejaculate. The fertility is hardly affected if the abnormal spermatozoa do not exceed 15-20%. There is a wide variation in the opinion regarding importance of varying degree of sperm abnormalities. However above 30-35% of total abnormalities are not suited to achieve good fertility. Most of the workers agree that semen of fertile bulls should not have more than 4% head abnormalities, 4-10% middle piece abnormalities, 5% tail abnormalities, 6% free heads and a total of 20% sperm abnormalities. Abnormalities associated with live spermatozoa are more important. The stain and technique used for the preparation of the stained smear are same as employed for live and dead count of the spermatozoa. Extended semen is not satisfactory for the morphological study of the spermatozoa because of the egg yolk or milk present in the dilutor. Sometimes the slide prepared is so concentrated with spermatozoa that it becomes difficult to observe individual spermatozoa. To overcome this problem, the semen samples may be diluted as per need (generally 1 : 5) with physiological saline solution. All glass slides used should be well cleaned, soaked in alcohol (to make them grease free) and dried. The normal spermatozoa consists of head, neck, middle piece and tail.

The detailed structure of the normal mammalian sperm cells is shown in Fig. 13.14. The spermatozoa have mainly three types of abnormalities viz. primary, secondary and tertiary.

Primary abnormalities are those that occur due to disorders of the seminiferous or germinal epithelium. **Secondary Abnormalities** are those that occur after the sperms have left the germinal epithelium during their passage through the efferent ducts, epididymis and vas deferens (Fig. 13.15). **Tertiary Abnormalities** are due to damage to the spermatozoa during or after ejaculation or during handling because of excessive agitation, overheating, too rapid cooling, presence of water and urine etc. In general, when in the semen sample, the percentage of primary and secondary abnormalities are high, the bull's fertility potential is low.

Primary abnormalities

These include :

1. Microcephalic head
2. Macrocephalic head
3. Elongated narrow head
4. Short broad head
5. Pyriform head
6. Double head
7. Double middle piece and tail
8. Abnormalities of the form of middle piece (e.g. swelling)
9. Abaxially attached middle piece
10. Highly coiled middle piece and tail

Secondary abnormalities

These include :

1. Detached normal heads
2. Proximal and distal protoplasmic droplets
3. Spermatozoa with bent tail
4. Detached and loosened galea capitis

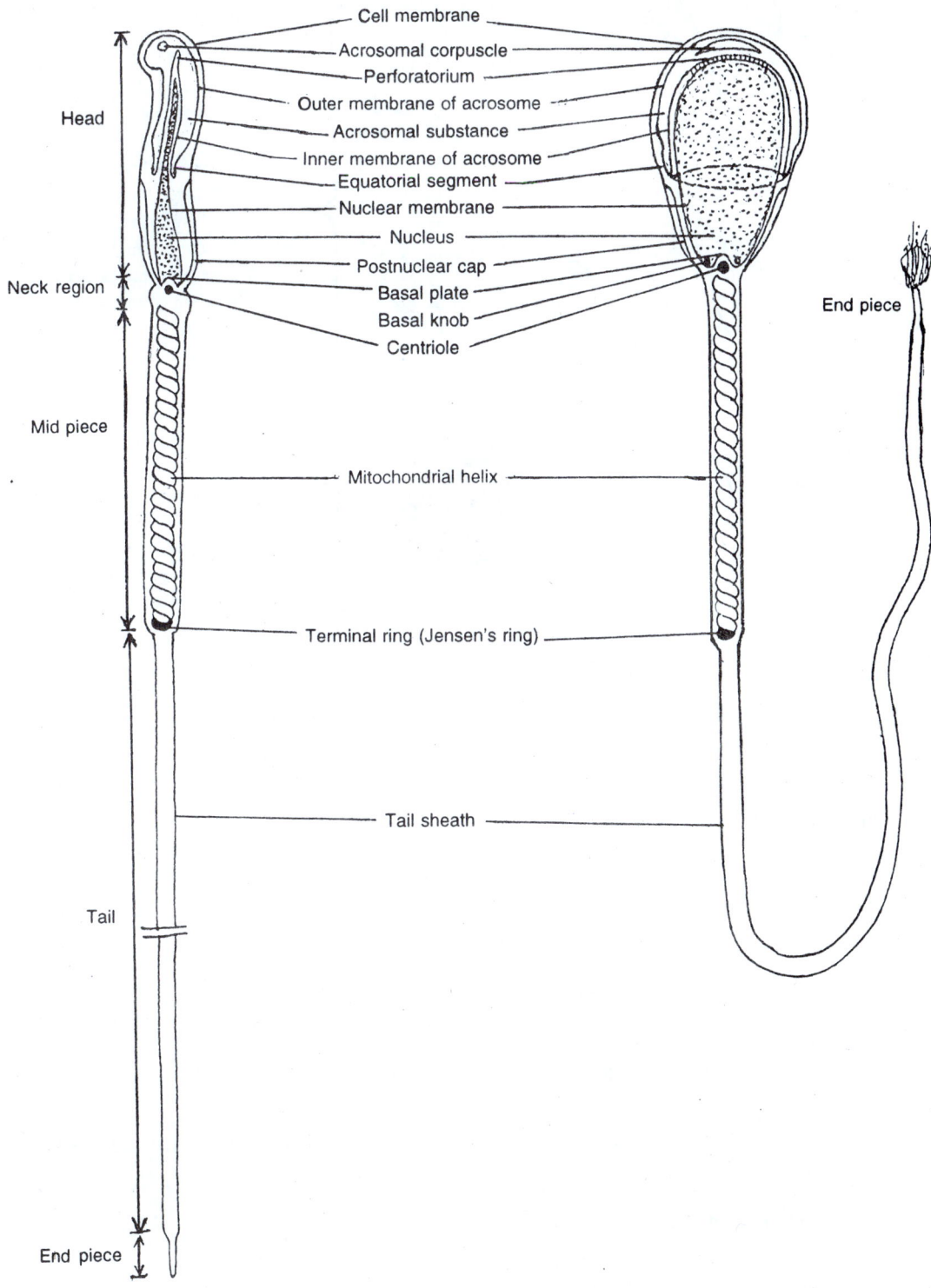

Head

Cell membrane
Acrosomal corpuscle
Perforatorium
Outer membrane of acrosome
Acrosomal substance
Inner membrane of acrosome
Equatorial segment
Nuclear membrane
Nucleus

Neck region

Postnuclear cap
Basal plate
Basal knob
Centriole

Mid piece

Mitochondrial helix

End piece

Terminal ring (Jensen's ring)

Tail sheath

Tail

End piece

Fig. 13.14. Detailed structure of normal mammalian sperm cell.

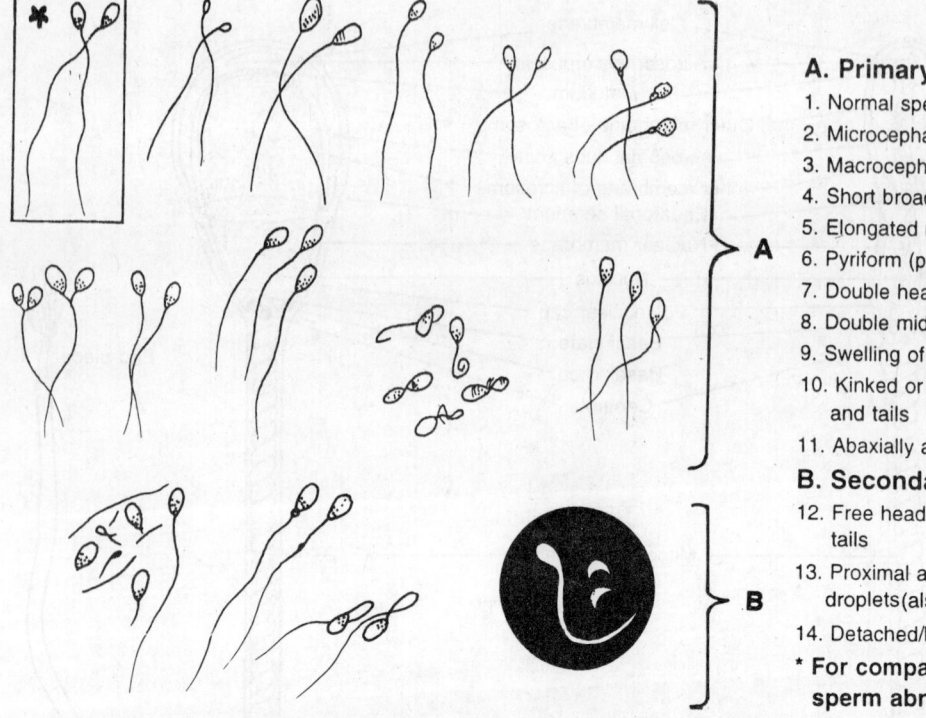

A. Primary

1. Normal sperm*
2. Microcephalic sperm
3. Macrocephalic sperm
4. Short broad head
5. Elongated narrow head
6. Pyriform (pear-shaped) head
7. Double heads
8. Double middle pieces and tails
9. Swelling of middle pieces
10. Kinked or coiled middle pieces and tails
11. Abaxially attached middle pieces

B. Secondary

12. Free heads, middle pieces and tails
13. Proximal and distal protoplasmic droplets(also bent middle pieces)
14. Detached/loosened galea capitis

* **For comparing different sperm abnormalities.**

Fig. 13.15. Sperm abnormalities.

Other cells found in semen smears

The different miscellaneous cells found in the semen are shown in Fig. 13.16.

1. Leukocytes because of infections in the reproductive tract
2. Erythrocytes
3. Squamous epithelial cells mostly from prepuce
4. Free floating protoplasmic droplets (have no significance)
5. Primordial spermiogenic cells
6. Spermatids
7. Spermatocytes
8. Medusa cells (These are portions from ciliated epithelium from the efferent ducts of testes. These cells have brush like projections. These cells are seen in great number in severe testicular hypoplasia.)
9. Giant or multinucleated cells seen in cases of testicular hypoplasia or degeneration
10. Degenerating sperm cell cluster. (Such clusters are seen in abundance in cases of testicular degeneration. Such degenerating clusters are produced due to disturbance in the spermatogenesis.)

Other tests for semen

1. Catalase test
2. Resistance to cold shock

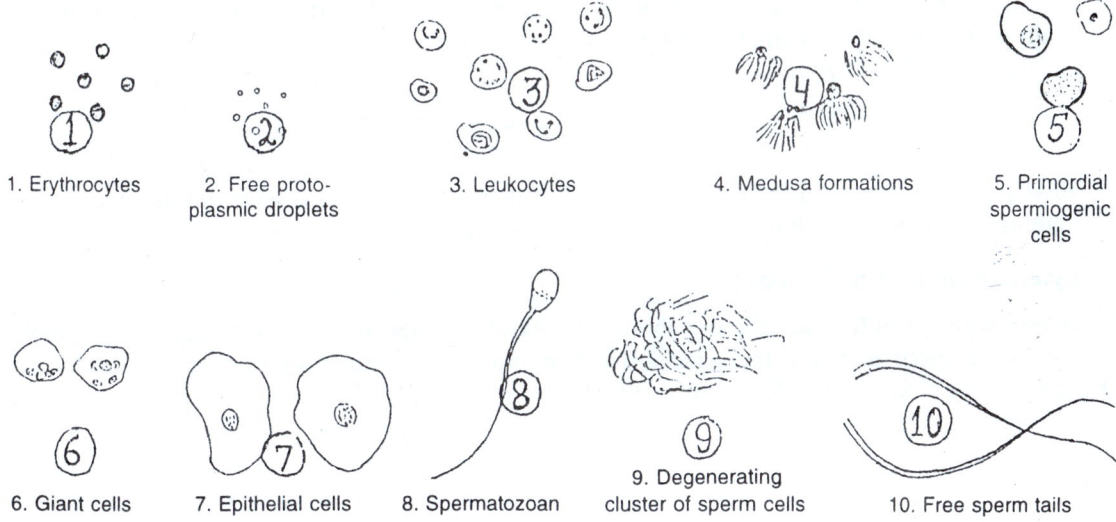

1. Erythrocytes   2. Free proto-plasmic droplets   3. Leukocytes   4. Medusa formations   5. Primordial spermiogenic cells

6. Giant cells   7. Epithelial cells   8. Spermatozoan   9. Degenerating cluster of sperm cells   10. Free sperm tails

Fig. 13.16. Miscellaneous cells found in semen.

3. Millovanov's resistance test (R-test)
4. Methylene blue reduction test
5. Resazurin reduction test
6. Fructolysis index
7. Oxygen utilization test

Catalase Test

The catalase test is not routinely carried out. This test may be carried out to detect increase in the catalase enzyme in the presence of pus and blood and the bacterial contamination in the semen.

Resistance to Cold Shock

This test is useful to test semen samples for varying degree of resistance of spermatozoa against cold shock. It may be likely that the semen having more spermatozoa with resistance against cold shock live longer when preserved and may predict high fertility.

Method

1. Take small quantity (0.25 to 0.5 ml) of undiluted semen in a small tube.
2. Immerse the tube in crushed ice (sudden change of temperature from 37°C to 0°C) and keep it for 10 minutes.
3. Remove the tube and thaw at 30°C.
4. Prepare slide in Eosin-Nigrosin stain for live and dead count.

Recovery of large number of live spermatozoa would mean better resistance against cold shock.

Millovanov's Resistance Test (R-test)

This test shows the ability of the spermatozoa to withstand 1% sodium chloride solution.

Method

1. Take 0.02 ml of freshly collected semen in 200 ml capacity flask.

2. Add 10 ml of 1% Sod. chloride solution in several steps and after each addition examine a drop of mixture under microscope till progressive motility of all the spermatozoa is ceased.

3. Calculate R-value (Resistance) as below :

$$R-value = \frac{ml \ of \ Sod. \ chloride \ solution \ required \ to \ cease \ the \ progressive \ motility}{0.02}$$

Good quality semen would have R-value not less than 5000 i.e. progressive motility wold cease after adding more than 100 ml of 1% Sod. chloride solution.

Methylene Blue Reduction Test

It is a very simple test to study the metabolic activity of the spermatozoa. As a result of metabolic activity of the spermatozoa in the semen, hydrogen ions are liberated under anaerobic condition. These hydrogen ions are transferred to methylene blue and the methylene blue is reduced to leuco methylene blue which is colourless. More are the number of the hydrogen ions liberated , less is the time taken by methylene blue for reduction and to change its blue color. The reduction time is directly related to the motility and the concentration of the spermatozoa in the semen sample.

Method

1. Add 0.2 ml of freshly collected semen in a small test tube containing 0.8 ml EYC (Egg Yolk Citrate) dilutor.

2. Add 0.1 ml of methylene blue solution in the above diluted semen and mix the contents (to prepare methylene blue solution, 50 mg of methylene blue is dissolved in 100 ml of 3% Sod. citrate dihydrate solution).

3. Seal the mixture by covering it with a 1 to 1.5 cm. thick layer of liquid paraffin or mineral oil to ensure anaerobic condition.

4. Place the tube containing the mixture in a water bath at 46.5°C.

5. Note the time taken for the disappearance of the blue colour.

A good quality semen would reduce the methylene blue in only 3-5 minutes. Average samples, would require about 9 minutes and poor samples would require > 9 minutes.

Resazurin Reduction Test

Like methylene blue reduction test, Rasazurin reduction test is also employed to evaluate the metabolic activity of semen based on the dehydrogenase activity of the spermatozoa. As a result of dehydrogenase enzyme activity in the sperm cells hydrogen ions are liberated which reduces Resazurin. Resazurin upon reduction undergoes a series of colour changes. Resazurin (blue) is first reduced to resurufin (pink) and finally to hydroresurufin (colorless).

Resazurin → Resurufin (irreversible)
(Blue)   (Pink)

Resurufin ↔ Hydroresurufin (reversible)
(Pink)   (Colourless)

Method

1. Add 0.2 ml of freshly collected undiluted semen in a small test tube.

2. Add 0.1 ml of Resazurin solution in the above undiluted semen and mix the contents (to prepare resazurin solution 5.5 mg of resazurin is dissolved in 100 ml distilled water).

3. Cover the mixture with 1 cm. thick layer of liquid paraffin or mineral oil to ensure anaerobic condition.
4. Incubate the contents at 45°C.
5. Look for change in colour i.e. blue to purple and from purple to colourless.

In good samples colour changes from :

Blue to pink or purple	1 minute
Pink to colourless	3-4 minutes

The average samples would take a time of about 5 minutes for second end point.

Fructolysis Index

It is described as the amount of fructose (mg) utilized by 10^9 spermatozoa in 1 hour at 37°C. Fructolysis has a direct correlation with the metabolic activity of the spermatozoa. This test is not a rapid test and is not of much practical value in routine semen evaluation work.

Oxygen Utilization Test

Oxygen is utilized for the oxidation of substrates outside the cell wall (exogenous respiration) and also for the oxidation of intracellular material (endogenous respiration). The measurement of oxygen uptake is related to the biochemical changes taking place in whole semen. If the spermatozoa are very active, they utilize more oxygen per unit of time. This test alone is not a dependable test for fertility and is not a test of routine practical value.

TESTS FOR THE EXAMINATION OF SPECIFIC INFECTIOUS DISEASES

The venereal or semen-borne diseases have a special concern in the examination for breeding soundness of bulls. The bulls should be tested periodically against *Brucellosis, Campylobacteriosis, Leptospirosis, Trichomoniasis, Tuberculosis* and Johne's disease (*Paratuberculosis*).

Chapter 14

Semen Collection

Hygienic collection of semen is an integral part of an artificial insemination programme. The following are the different methods of semen collection in **bull**.

1. Directly from vagina after natural service by means of a spoon or syringe with a long nozzle.
2. By rectal massage of the ampullae of vas deferens and seminal vesicles per rectum.
3. By electro-ejaculation.
4. Using artificial vagina (A.V.).

DIRECTLY FROM VAGINA AFTER NATURAL SERVICE

This is the simplest and oldest method of semen collection. After a natural service of the cow, the semen is collected from vagina using either a long spoon or a syringe with long nozzle. Good quality semen cannot be obtained by this method, since the semen is always mixed with large volume of mucus.

BY RECTAL MASSAGE OF THE AMPULLAE OF THE VAS DEFERENS AND SEMINAL VESICLES

It is an useful method for bulls which are lame or are unwilling or are unable to copulate. There are certain restraints for efficient semen collection through this techniques e.g.

(a) Some skill and experience is necessary to massage ampullae and the seminal vesicles per rectum.

(b) Some bulls respond poorly to this method of semen collection.

(c) Because the semen dribbles through preputial hairs, semen collection is not clean.

(d) The massage of ampullae sometimes stimulates urination.

The bull is securely restrained in a service crate. Hand with full arm obstetrical rubber sleeve after lubrication is inserted in the rectum and feces is evacuated. The seminal vesicles are massaged pressing towards urthera for few minutes. Simultaneously an assistant is kept ready to collect semen as it drips. Then the ampullae are massaged and milked one by one and are stripped off by pressing against the floor of the pelvis. The pelvic urethra may also be massaged. Prior stimulation with a cow may be of great help in collecting semen through massage technique. After the massage of the ampullae the S-curve of the penis should be straightened to allow escape of semen, if retained in sigmoid flexure. There are chances that if massaged regularly, the bulls may become accustomed with this technique within 3-4 weeks.

ELECTRO-EJACULATION

The electro-ejaculation method is rarely used for semen collection in bulls. The method is painful to bulls. The electro-ejaculation method of semen collection may be used in valuable and crippled bulls that cannot mount and also in old bulls which have no desire to mount. In this method, weak and alternating current is provided to sacral and pelvic nerves with the electrode placed in the rectum. Depending upon the size of the bull, various sizes of the electrodes (diameter ranging from 4.0-8.0 cm and length ranging from 35.0 to 60.0 cm) are available. The preputial hairs may be clipped and the adjacent area washed, rinsed and properly dried. Sexual stimulation with a cow or rectal manipulation of the ampullae and seminal vesicles prior to electro-ejaculation would greatly aid in collecting good semen sample. The bull should be fastened in strong stanchion. The footing should be non-slippery. The probe after being lubricated with non-insulating lubricant is inserted about 30.0-45.0 cm into the rectum and is held from outside anus on the middle against the ventral floor of the pelvis. A gradually increasing alternating current (from 0-5 volts) is passed which is later gradually reduced (5 volts to 0) in 5-10 seconds. Current frequencies may range from 15 to 90 cycles/second. Subsequent stimulations are slowly increased. Erection and ejaculation occurs at 10-15 volts when 0.5-1.0 ampere current is flowing. Excessive stimulation at higher voltage may cause a degree of ataxia or the bull may fall down. With electro-ejaculation it takes about 3-5 minutes for semen collection. Though there is no difference in the percentage of motile, live or abnormal spermatozoa, the concentration and the total number of sperms per ejaculate are low with electro-ejaculation compared to collection with artificial vagina.

THE ARTIFICIAL VAGINA METHOD

This is the most widely accepted method of semen collection.. Through A.V. a complete and clean ejaculate is promptly obtained. The best time of semen collection is early morning before feeding. In the morning hours, the bulls are fresh and alert. Bulls may become reluctant to donate semen in full belly after feeding. If semen is collected early in a day, it can be utilized the same day also and this may help achieving higher fertility. The bull, prior to semen collection should be properly cleaned. Clipping of preputial hairs should be done occasionally. Preputial region may be thoroughly washed and dried. The attendants, leading the bulls, should be well acquainted to the bull. The dummy should also be well clean and dry. It should be strong enough to sustain the weight and thrust of the bull. The dummy should be of docile nature and of appropriate size. The tail of dummy should be tied to one side. All the parts of A.V. must be thoroughly clean, dry and sterile before being assembled. The different parts of the AV are shown in Fig. 14.1 and include :

1. Heavy rubber cylinder
2. Inner rubber lining
3. Rubber cone
4. Graduated semen collection tube
5. Insulating bag
6. Valve

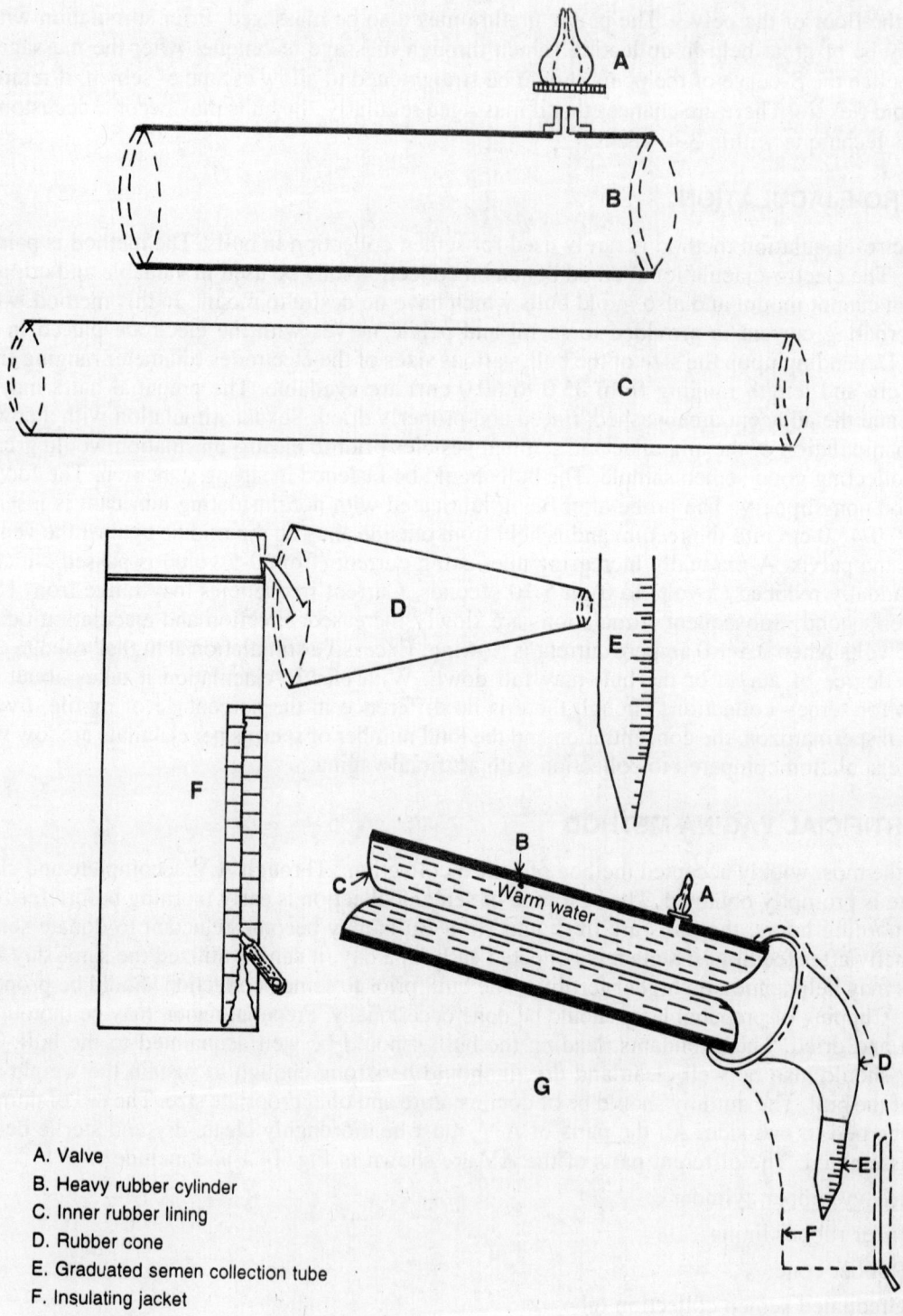

A. Valve
B. Heavy rubber cylinder
C. Inner rubber lining
D. Rubber cone
E. Graduated semen collection tube
F. Insulating jacket
G. Assembled A.V.

Fig. 14.1. Different parts of A.V. and assembled A.V.

The heavy rubber cylinder is made up of hard rubber. It is approximately 8.0-10.0 cm. in diameter and 35.0-40.0 cm. in length. The outer edges of the heavy rubber cylinder are upturned so as to provide a firm grip with inner rubber lining. There is a hole at about 5.0 cm from one end to which a valve is attached. Through this hole hot water is introduced or removed to warm the artificial vagina at a fixed temperature. The hard rubber cylinder is fitted with an inner rubber lining which is longer enough than the length of the hard rubber cylinder. Rough surfaced inner rubber liner is preferred by bulls compared to smooth surface rubber liner. This inner rubber lining having a diameter of 7.0-7.2 cm is turned back over the two ends of the hard rubber cylinder and is tightly held in place by thick rubber bands. A rubber cone of about 20.00 cm length is fitted to the valve end of the AV. To the narrow end of the cone is fitted a clean and sterilized graduated semen collection tube. The graduated semen collection tube and the rubber cone are covered with an insulating jacket.

For proper thrust and ejaculatory reflex, it is important that the proper temperature and pressure be maintained in the artificial vagina along with proper lubrication. The bulls may refuse semen ejaculation in an AV which is either too hot or too cold. The bulls donate semen at 39 to 41°C depending upon the liking of the bull. Firstly hot water of about 70°C is added through the inlet of the cylinder. This water is then drained out. This is done as a measure for prewarming the AV to avoid sudden fall in temperature of warm water which is added later to obtain the requisite temperature (39-41°C). Temperatures above 45°C may kill sperms and also the bulls may refuse to serve at higher temperatures. Very low temperatures may also fail to induce ejaculatory response. Sterilized and neutral white vaseline is non-toxic to spermatozoa and is used for lubrication. Care should be taken to use lubrication to its minimum so as to avoid trickling down of the lubricants in the semen collection tube. The first 7-8 cm opening of the A.V. should be lightly lubricated for easy introduction of the penis.

Proper pressure of the A.V. is also important to stimulate ejaculatory response. Pressure is maintained by inflating air through the vent till such time that the thumb may easily be inserted in to the lumen of the A.V.

Steps in Semen Collection

1. Secure dummy in a service crate and tie its tail to one side.
2. Collector should stand on right side of the dummy.
3. Prior teasing of bull e.g. showing to other mounting bulls, restraining for few minutes prior to collection and allowing mounting and then forcing to dismount helps in obtaining complete ejaculate.
4. Again allow the bull to mount. Direct the penis in the A.V. Left hand of the collector may be used to direct the penis in A.V. by putting the left palm under the sheath.
5. The bull donates semen with a thrust. The A.V. Is kept on the penis while the bull is dismounting after thrust.
6. After semen collection the A.V. is held vertically to allow the semen to drain completely into the semen collection tube.
7. The semen collection tube is withdrawn from the A.V. This is kept well protected from light and temperature shock. It is marked for identification, corked or covered and is put in a water bath at 35-37°C.

Chapter 15

Preservation of Semen at Ambient and Refrigeration Temperatures

PRECAUTIONS

For extending (diluting) semen, the following precautions should be adopted.

1. Dilutors should be prepared aseptically with analytical grade chemicals.
2. Pure substances and clean and sterilized equipments should be used.
3. Handling of semen should be done carefully to avoid cold shock, overheating and contamination with urine, dust and water, exposure to direct sunlight and excessive agitation etc.

BASIC PREREQUISITES (BASIC PRINCIPLES) OF SEMEN DILUTION

The basic prerequisites of satisfactory diluents for semen preservation are :

1. Maintaining proper osmotic pressure of approximately 300 milliosmoles (which is equivalent to blood, semen and milk).
2. Provision for buffering substances to maintain a nearly neutral pH.
3. Provision for nutrients for both aerobic and anaerobic metabolic processes.
4. Provision for protection against cold shock (e.g. Lecithin in egg yolk, phospholipids in milk and glycerol in deep freezing).
5. Antibiotics to cover broad range of bacteria.

The semen dilutors can be categorized into three groups as :

1. Diluents for the preservation of semen at room temperature (Ambient temperature—18 to 30°C).
   (a) Coconut Milk Extender (CME)
   (b) Millovanov's dilutor
   (c) Illini Variable Temperature (IVT) dilutor
2. Dilutents for the preservation of semen at refrigeration temperature (4-5°C)
   (a) Egg Yolk Citrate (EYC)
   (b) D_2 dilutor

    (c) Milk dilutor

    (d) Kampschmidit's dilutor

    (e) Egg yolk phosphate dilutor

3. Diluents for the preservation of semen at sub zero temperature (–79 to –196°C)

4. Glycerolated Egg yolk citrate dilutor

5. Milk glycerol dilutor

6. Egg yolk tris dilutor

COMPOSITION OF DIFFERENT DILUTORS

Diluents for the preservation of semen at room temperature (Ambient temperature 18 to 30°C)

Coconut Milk Extender (CME)

(A) Buffer, Antibiotics and Catalase

(a)	Sodium citrate dihydrate	2.2 gm
(b)	Penicillin G. Sodium	60.0 mg
(c)	Dihydrostreptomycin sulfate	135.0 mg
(d)	Sulfanilamide	300.0 mg
(e)	Polymyxin B sulfate	10.0 mg
(f)	Aqueous solution of catalase	15,000 units
(g)	Mycostatin	1,000 units
(h)	Glass distilled water	60-70 ml

(B) Coconut Milk : Boil the coconut water for 10 min and filter it. Add 15 ml of coconut milk (water) to section **(A)**.

(C) Add 7 ml of **egg yolk** to the solution **(A)** + **(B)**. Bring the volume to 100 ml using distilled water. Adjust the pH to 7.4 with 10% NaOH solution.

Preservation of semen in CME at room temperature (18-30°C) maintains motility and fertility satisfactorily for 3-4 days. The vials should be filled completely to avoid air space and should be stored in a dark place. Exposure to light should be avoided. Due to non-availability of good equality of coconut water round the year and in all regions of the country its use has not been commercialized.

Millovanov's Dilutor

Part A

1.	Pot. dihydrogen phosphate	72 mg
2.	Distilled water	10 ml

Part B

1.	Sod. citrate dihydrate	2.025 gm
2.	Glucose	0.570 gm
3.	Sod. bicarbonate	0.125 gm
4.	Penicillin G. Sodium	60.000 mg
5.	Dihydrostreptomycin sulfate	0.100 gm

6. Sulphanilamide   0.300 gm
7. Glass distilled water   90.000 ml

Mix part **A** and part **B** in the ratio of 1 : 9.

(C) Add 11 ml of **egg yolk** to the above solution **(A) + (B)**.

Illini Variable Temperature (IVT) dilutor

The dilutor consists of :

1. Sod. citrate dihydrate   2.000 gm
2. Sod. bicarbonate   0.210 gm
3. Pot. chloride   0.040 gm
4. Glucose   0.300 gm
5. Sulphamilamide   0.300 gm
6. Distilled water   100 ml

Carbon dioxide gas is passed (bubbled) through the above solution until the pH reaches to 6.3. Egg yolk is mixed at 10% level. Streptomycin and Penicillin are added @ of 1000 μg and 1000 I.U. per ml, respectively.

The diluted semen is stored in 1 ml ampoules at room temperature. Ampoules should be flushed with CO_2 immediately before filling. As little air space as possible should be left inside the ampoules.

Diluents for the preservation of semen at refrigeration temperature

Egg Yolk Citrate (EYC) Dilutor

1. Sod. citrate dihydrate   2.9 gm
2. Penicillin G. Sodium   1 lac units
3. Dihydrostreptomycin sulfate   100 mg
4. Sulfanilamide   300 mg
5. Distilled water   added to 100 ml

20% of the egg yolk is added in the above buffer solution. To prepare 100 ml of EYC dilutor 20 ml of Egg yolk is added to 80 ml of the above citrate buffer solution. Sod. citrate disperses the fat globules in the yolk in such a way that individual spermatozoa can be observed clearly under the microscope.This dilutor is very popular for bull semen dilution and semen remains fit for insemination for 3-4 days. However, for buffalo semen it does not keep on well for more than 2 days.

Collection of egg yolk : Fresh unfertilized chicken eggs are used for the collection of egg yolk to be used in semen dilutor. Egg surface is cleaned with 70% alcohol soaked in cotton. The egg shell is cracked at the pointed end with the help of sterilized forceps. A hole is made in the egg shell by removing cracked shell. The albumin is allowed to pour out in a beaker. The hole size is increased and the yolk ball is collected gently on sterilized filter paper. The yolk ball is gently rolled on filter paper to remove albumin. The yolk ball membrane is gently punctured with a sterilized object and yolk is collected in sterilized graduated cylinder.

D$_2$ dilutor

1. Sod. bicarbonate (1.3% solution)   10 parts
2. Glucose (5% solution)   40 parts
3. Fructose (5% solution)   25 parts
4. Egg yolk   25 parts

One lac units of Penicillin G. Sodium and 100 mg of Dihydrostreptomycin sulfate are added to 100 ml of D$_2$ dilutor before use.

Kampschmidt's dilutor

1. Dextrose (5%)   4 parts
2. Sod. bicarbonate (1.3%)   1 part
3. Sulphamezathine (2%)   1 part
4. Egg yolk   1 part

Penicillin G. Sodium (1 lac units) and dihydrostreptomycin sulfate (100 mg) should be added to 100 ml of above dilutor.

Milk dilutor

- Take homogenized or skimmed pasteurized milk. Skim milk is preferred as it has few or no fat globules to interfere with microscopic examination of semen.
- Heat to 92-95°C for 10 min in a Pyrex glass boiler.
- Cool to room temperature.
- Pour down the milk from the boiler leaving the surface scum of albumin on the sides of the boiler.
- Add following :

  Sulphanilamide   0.3 gm/ml
  Penicillin G. Sodium   1000 units/ml
  Dihydrostreptomycin sulphate   1000 µg/ml

Milk as such contains a spermicidal factor, lactanin. The protective fraction of the milk is composed of phospholipids. The toxic fraction of milk (lactanin) is removed with the removal of albumin from milk.

Egg-Yolk Phosphate Dilutor

Part A

Disodium hydrogen phosphate   2.0 gm
Pot. dihydrogen phosphate   0.2 gm
Distilled water   added to 100 ml

Part B

Egg yolk.

Mix equal parts of phosphate buffer solution (**A**) and egg yolk (**B**).

Bull semen can be preserved at 5°C for 72 to 96 hours. Buffalo semen keeps on well up to 48 hours.

Note : The diluents for preservation of semen at subzero temperature (–79°C to –196°C) are discussed in Chapter 17 (Deep Freezing of Semen).

Chapter 16

Semen Dilution

The semen dilution is done basically with the following two objectives :

1. To increase number of services of the females from one ejaculate of the male.
2. To maintain the viability of the sperms during storage period.

The semen is extended to such an appropriate volume so that each inseminating dose of semen contains sufficient number of motile spermatozoa needed for optimum fertility. The volume and the number of the spermatozoa needed per dose of insemination in different species are given in Table 16.1.

Table 16.1. Volume of semen and No. of spermatozoa required for A.I. with frozen and liquid semen

Dose	Frozen semen		Liquid semen			
	In ampoules (for cattle)	In straws (for cattle)	Cattle	Sheep	Swine	Horse
Volume (ml)	1.00	0.25 to 0.5	1.0	0.2	50.0	30.0 to 50.0
No. of motile spermatozoa (millions)	15	15	10	50	2000	500

The following should be ensured before dilution.

1. All sterilized glasswares and other articles are assembled on the working bench in advance.
2. Semen and the dilutor are maintained at equal temperature.

As a precaution, small quantity of the dilutor may be added slowly to the few drops of the semen.If this is maintained satisfactorily, the whole semen may be extended. This would save the semen, in case the dilutor is not fit for sperm survival due to any mistake at any step. After initial checking the dilution of the semen should be done in two steps. The first step dilution is done immediately after semen collection and its initial examination. The second step (final) dilution should be done after detailed semen examination and assessing the final dilution rate so that each dose of insemination contains minimum number of normal and motile spermatozoa for optimum fertility.

Example for semen dilution for EYC dilutor (liquid semen)

Let

Volume of ejaculate = 4.0 ml

Density/ml = 1200×10^6

Motile spermatozoa 70%

Calculation for dilution

$$1 \text{ ml of semen contains } \frac{1200 \times 10^6 \times 70}{100} = 840 \times 10^6 \text{ motile sperms}$$

The required dose of liquid semen is 1 ml and the number of the motile sperms required is 10×10^6 per insemination

$$\text{Hence the dilution rate is } \frac{840 \times 10^6}{10 \times 10^6} = 84$$

Hence 4 ml of the semen may be diluted to $(4 \times 84 \text{ ml}) = 336$ ml

When such a high number of doses are not required for inseminating the cows, the dilution rate may be reduced.

Note : In case of frozen semen 20-80% spermatozoa are killed during freezing and hence the dilution rate is reduced depending upon the expectancy of spermatozoa losses (based on trials) and the dose of frozen semen (straws have 0.25 to 0.5 ml semen, and the ampoules have 1.0 ml semen).

The liquid semen should be stored in sterilized glass vials or tubes. The vials/tubes should be filled completely to leave minimum possible space for air. The presence of air causes more jolts during transportation. The processed semen should be protected from sudden cooling and cold shock. The semen vials/tubes should be labeled properly for identity e.g.

1. Name, number and breed of the bull.
2. Dilutor and dilution rate.
3. Date of semen collection.

Chapter 17

Deep Freezing of Semen

In deep freezing of semen the metabolic processes of the spermatozoa are arrested to its least and negligible amounts of waste products are formed. Resistance to deep freezing of the spermatozoa varies from species to species and from individual to individual. Nearly 50% spermatozoa (range 20 to 80%) are lost in the deep freezing process. Bull speprmatooa are very sensitive to cold shock. The amount of dilution in deep freezing is so determined that after freezing and thawing there should remain 8 to 12 million actively motile spermatozoa per dose of frozen semen. Glycerol is the universally used cryprotectant in the deep freezing of the spermatozoa. Glycerol minimizes the formation of ice crystals within spermatozoa. Considerable amount of water is attached to glycerol, when added in the medium and thus least water is made available for ice crystal formation. When glycerol is not added in the dilutor, there is formation of ice crystals which expand more and more and thus the spermatozoa are compressed. When glycerol is added in the dilutor, the size of crystal is much smaller and there are channels in between crystals, in which spermatozoa lie without being compressed. In the absence of glycerol, as a result of extra and intracellular crystallization of water, salts in residual fluid get concentrated, the residual fluid becomes hypertonic and spermatozoa are put under extreme osmotic stress.

DILUENTS FOR PRESERVATION OF SEMEN AT SUBZERO TEMPERATURE

The commonly used dilutors for the preservation of semen at subzero temperature are glycerolated eggs yolk citrate dilutor, milk glycerol dilutor and egg yolk tris dilutor.

Glycerolated Egg Yolk Citrate Dilutor

The EYC dilutor is prepared as described earlier for preservation of semen at refrigeration temperature except that sulphanilamide is not added.

Note : Sulphanilamide crystallizes during freezing process causing damage to spermatozoa and hence its use is not recommended in dilutors for deep freezing of semen.

1. Sod. citrate dihydrate   2.9 gm
2. Penicillin G. Sodium   1 lac units
3. Dihydrostreptomycin sulfate   100 mg
4. Distilled water   added to 100 ml

The dilutor is prepared in two parts, A and B.

A-part : Nothing is added to part A.

B-part : Glycerol is added @ 14%.

Method

(a) Assess the final dilution rate and dilute the semen to the extent of 50% only of the final dilution in part A of the dilutor.

(b) Store the diluted semen (A) and glycerated dilutor (14% glycerol) i.e. part (B) for 4 hrs. at refrigeration temp. (5°C).

(c) Complete the remaining 50% dilution with part-B having 14% glycerol at 5°C.

The second half (part B) of the dilutor should be added in 4 equal amounts at 20 min interval or should be added drop wise so that the entire part-B is added in 1 hr. period.

(d) Leave the mixture (semen + part-A + part-B) for 12 hrs. at 5°C for equilibration before freezing. This is known as equilibration period.

Note : Equilibration time is the period needed by sperm cells prior to freezing to become adjusted with the dilutor so that excessive loss of spermatozoa does not occur during the freezing process. With equilibration time, the spermatozoa cell membrane may become more permeable and the spermatozoa may withstand critical temperature (−15 to −25°C) much better. Different workers have suggested different times (ranging from 1/2 to 18 hrs.) for equilibration. Addition of sugars like fructose and arabinose helps in reducing equilibration time. Presently earlier recommendation of 15 to 18 hrs. for equilibration time are generally not followed and the equilibration time of 4-6 hrs. appears practical. Neither the post-thaw motility nor the fertility is affected by such reduction in the equilibration time.

Milk Glycerol Dilutor

The dilutor is prepared in the same way as described earlier under dilutors for refrigeration temperature. As for other dilutors for deep freezing sulfanilamide is not added in the dilutor. The glycerol is mixed in steps as described for glycerolated egg yolk citrate dilutor. Equilibration time is also needed for sperm cells before freezing to become adjusted to the dilutor.

Glycerolated Egg Yolk Tris (EYT) Dilutor

1. Tris buffer (Tris hydroxymethyl) aminomethane;   3.028 gm
   2-Amino-2-(hydroxymethyl) propane-1,3-diol
2. Citric acid (monohydrate)   1.675 gm
3. Fructose (anhydrous)   1.250 gm
4. Glycerol   7 ml
5. Penicillin G. Sodium   1 lac units

6. Dihydrostreptomycin sulfate   100 mg
7. Glass distilled water   upto 100 ml

10 parts of egg yolk are mixed with 90 parts of buffer.

Inclusion of glycerol at room temperature is found as satisfactory as at 5°C. Tris dilutor allows filling and sealing of polyvinyl-chloride straws at room temperature while freezing the semen.

METHODS OF DEEP FREEZING

Using Glass Ampoules
Method

1. Immediately after equilibration, the semen is filled in previously marked ampoules.
2. Seal the ampoules over flame leaving about 0.5 ml air space.
3. Place the ampoules in ethyl alcohol or acetone bath at 5°C.
4. By adding small pieces of solid carbon dioxide (dry ice), bring the temperate from 5°C to −15°C at the rate of 1-2°C cooling per minute. Temperature is noted with dial thermometer.
5. When temperature is brought to −15°C the cooling rate is increased. The temperature is brought down by adding solid carbondioxide to −79°C at the rate of 4-5°C cooling per minute.
6. Ampoules of frozen semen are maintained in dry ice (−79°C) or in liquid nitrogen (−196°C). Liquid nitrogen storage of spermatozoa is better.

Note : Freezing semen in glass ampoules has become out of date now.

Using Polyvinyl Chloride Straws

Freezing of semen in polyvinyl chloride straws has gained popularity all over the world, because they require less storage space, have better freezing characteristics and are labelled, filled and sealed automatically. There is also minimum loss of spermatozoa during AI. Various types of the polyvinyl chloride straws are available in the market for freezing of semen. The common types are French medium straws/midi straws, French mini straws and conventional straws/mini tubes (Fig. 17.1). The approximate volume of semen within each straw, length of the straw and the approximate surface area of the straw are given in Table 17.1.

Table 17.1. Volume, length and surface area of various straws used in deep freezing of semen

Type of straw	Volume (ml)	Length (mm)	Surface area (mm^2)
French medium/midi straws	0.50	133	1152
French mini straws	0.25	133	823
Continental straws/mini tubes	0.25	65	555

The French medium and French mini straws have at one end two pieces of synthetic cotton/thread and polyvinyl alcohol powder placed in between them. The powder becomes gelatinous when comes in contact with semen. After filling the straw with semen the other end is sealed with polyvinyl alcohol powder. The continental straws (mini tubes) are sealed with steel/glass balls. The balls seal the straw perfectly well and no leakage occurs.

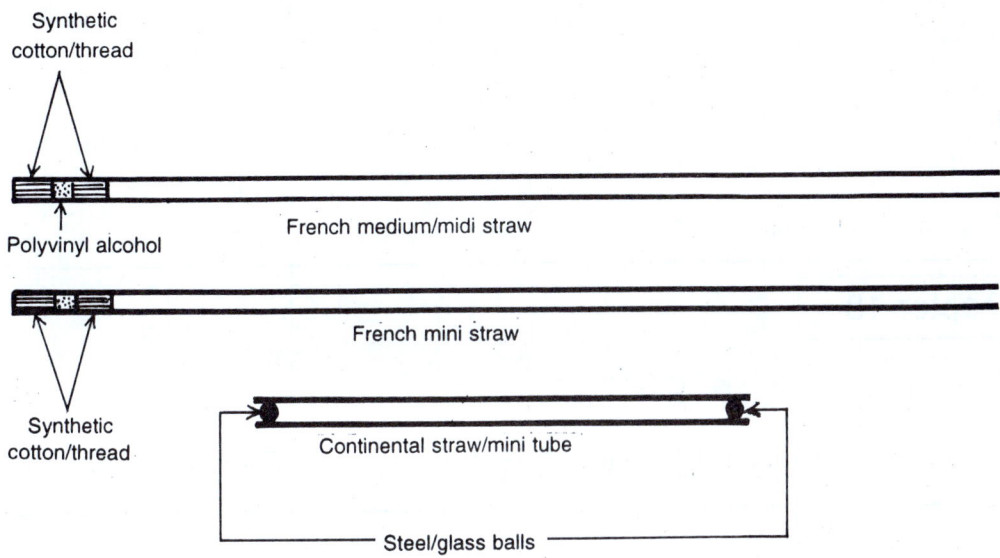

Fig. 17.1. Various types of straws used in cryopreservation of semen.

Method

1. Immediately after equilibration, the semen is filled in previously marked polyvinyl chloride straws. While using glycerolated Egg Yolk Tris (EYT) dilutor, mixing of glycerol in the buffer and also filling and sealing of straws may be done at room temperature and the sealed straws may be put for equilibration.

2. Equilibrated straws are dried in cold cabinet using absorbent material and are horizontally spread over a tray having bottom made of mesh wire to allow free movement of liquid nitrogen vapour.

3. The tray with straws is put in the liquid nitrogen tank over grill in a way that straws are about 4 cm. above the level of liquid nitrogen. At the level of straws the vapor temprature is about –175 to –180°C.

4. The liquid nitrogen tank is covered with lid.

5. The straws are left in the liquid nitrogen vapors for about 10 minutes.

6. The straws are collected and are placed in a goblet filled with liquid nitrogen in the nitrogen tank itself.

7. The goblet containing the frozen semen straws in liquid nitrogen is put in a canister and the canister is immersed in liquid nitrogen (–196°C).

Chapter 18

A.I. Techniques Using Chilled and Frozen Semen

Good quality semen, proper handling of semen, sound reproductive health of the cow, general hygiene and A.I. at proper time are must to obtain high fertility rates. The latter is extremely important.

CHECK POINTS BEFORE INSEMINATION

1. If the animal to be inseminated is heifer, check its body weight, At first service, the body weight should not be less than 240-250 kg in cattle heifers and 300 kg in buffalo heifers.
2. There should not be any abnormal discharge from genital organs.
3. The animal should not be a problem breeder. The problem breeders should be thoroughly examined and treated first.
4. Is there any chance for animal being pregnant? Such doubts should always be clarified by carrying out pregnancy diagnosis before performing A.I.
5. In case of any doubt for animal being not in heat, it should be examined thoroughly.
6. There should be a gap period of about 60 days after normal calving and of about 90 days after abnormal calving (e.g. Retained placenta, Abortion, Dystocia etc.).
7. The type of semen (Breed, No./Name of the bull and percentage of exotic blood etc.) should be decided in advance. The crossbred progeny should not have more than 62.5% exotic blood.

If above things are not checked prior to handling of semen for A.I., there are chances that either the semen may go waste or there may be problems during calving.

AI WITH LIQUID SEMEN

The sterilized catheter of about 40-42 cm. length, having outer diameter of 5-6 mm and inside diameter of about 1 mm is fitted to a clean and dry plastic or glass syringe (capacity 2 to 5 ml) with rubber connector. After sucking some air (0.5 to 1.0 ml) about 1 ml of the liquid semen is sucked in the pipette. Prior sucking of air(before semen) aids in complete expulsion the semen. The A.I. is done by recto-vaginal method.

Recto-vaginal Method of A.I.

1. Artificial insemination in cattle and buffalo is done in standing animals. The animals must be properly secured in the service crate.

2. The free hand and arm encased in obstetrical rubber sleeve, after lubrication is inserted into the rectum and after removing dung, the cervix is grasped. Care should be taken to prevent ballooning of rectum. If ballooning occurs, the cervix may be grasped after some time when the gas from the rectum has evacuated.

3. The vulva and the vulvar lips are carefully wiped with clean cotton. If necessary, the vulva and the perineal region may be thoroughly washed with clean water and then wiped dry with the help of clean absorbent cotton or towel.

4. While grasping the cervix with palm and fingers, the external os is guided with the help of thumb. The vulvar lips are pulled apart with the help of assistant and the inseminating catheter or A.I. gun is passed at an angle of 45° through vagina. In case the vaginal folds create problems and put hinderance for passing of catheter/A.I. gun, the cervix may be pushed forward to straighten the vagina and to abolish vaginal folds.

5. The A.I. catheter/A.I. gun is manipulated so as to strike thumb placed over the external os and then the catheter/A.I. gun is passed into the cervix. The catheter/A.I. gun by manipulation is passed about middle or two-third of the distance of the cervical length, where the semen is deposited slowly (Fig. 18.1).

6. After depositing semen in the cervix, catheter/A.I. gun is drawn out together with the arm in rectum.

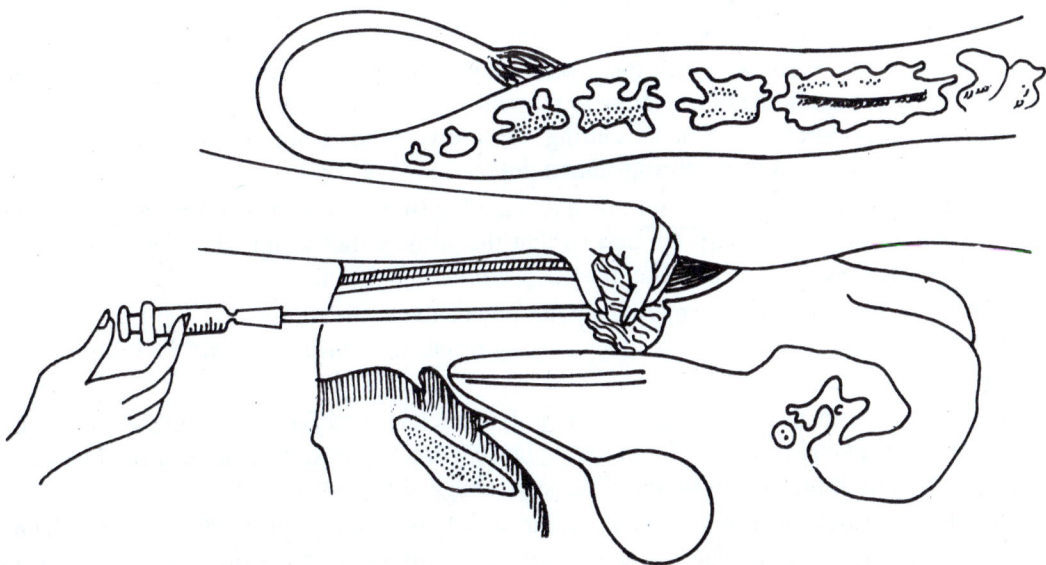

Fig. 18.1. Rectovaginal technique of inseminating cow.

Note : The semen should be deposited in the cervix only. Intrauterine inseminations should be avoided. There are chances of uterine diseases with intrauterine inseminations and abortion, if the animal is pregnant. Further, excessive manipulations and trauma to the cervix be avoided. If there is difficulty in passing the catheter, pass it as far as possible. Sometimes, especially in inseminating heifers, catheters with small diameters are easy to pass.

AI WITH FROZEN SEMEN

Using polyvinyl chloride straws

1. Be prepared. All necessary equipments should be ready at hand before opening the liquid nitrogen container. Frozen spermatozoa after thawing do not survive long and also they cannot be refrozen. The frozen semen once taken out from the LN_2 container, should be used soon after thawing.

2. Be sure about the desired semen and the identity of the canister in which it is kept.

3. Raise the desired canister to the neck of the container, keeping the straws in goblet as deep as possible. The canister should be raised only to the level from where the straws can be grasped (Fig. 18.2). Take out the desired straw/straws as quickly as possible and put them immediately in the thaw bath. Not more than 2-3 straws should be taken out at one time. The canister with goblets containing semen straws should remain in the neck of the LN_2 container for *shortest possible period* (few seconds only).

4. Thawing has been successfully done at temperatures ranging from ice water to nearly 70°C. At higher temperature, the percentage of motile spermatozoa and also the normal acrosome retention is higher, but thaw time must be carefully controlled to avoid killing of the spermatozoa due to over-heating. For straws thawing temperature of 35 to 37°C for 0.5 to 1 min. is recommended under field conditions. The thawing water should be fresh and clean (Fig. 18.3).

5. After thawing period, remove the straws from the water bath and wipe out all the water from the outer surface of the straw with an absorbent material.

6. Hold the straw vertically with the cotton plug (manufacturer's) downward. Shake the air bubble from the middle of the straw to the sealed end of the straw(not the factory seal). This location is important so that on cutting the straw, there is no loss of semen and there is continuous flow of semen during semen deposition (Fig. 18.4).

7. Cut the straw at right angle to remove the seal plug (not the manufacturer's plug) (Fig. 18.5). The scissors must be sharp enough so that the straw is not crimped. A sharply cut semen straw would securely fit into the plastic inseminating sheath.

8. Withdraw the piston (wire) of A.I. gun and place the straw in the chamber of A.I. gun. The manufacturer's plug should go inside the gun and the cut end should face out side (Fig. 18.6).

9. Take out the sheath from the container (polythene bag) and fix the sheath over the A.I. gun from its broad end (Figs. 18.7 and 18.8). The cut end of the semen straw should be securely fit to the top of the sheath to avoid semen leakage (Fig. 18.8).

10. Set the ring (lock) securely over the plastic sheath by pushing it forcefully against the broad portion of the A.I. gun. The sheath is a device which retains the straw and allows escape of

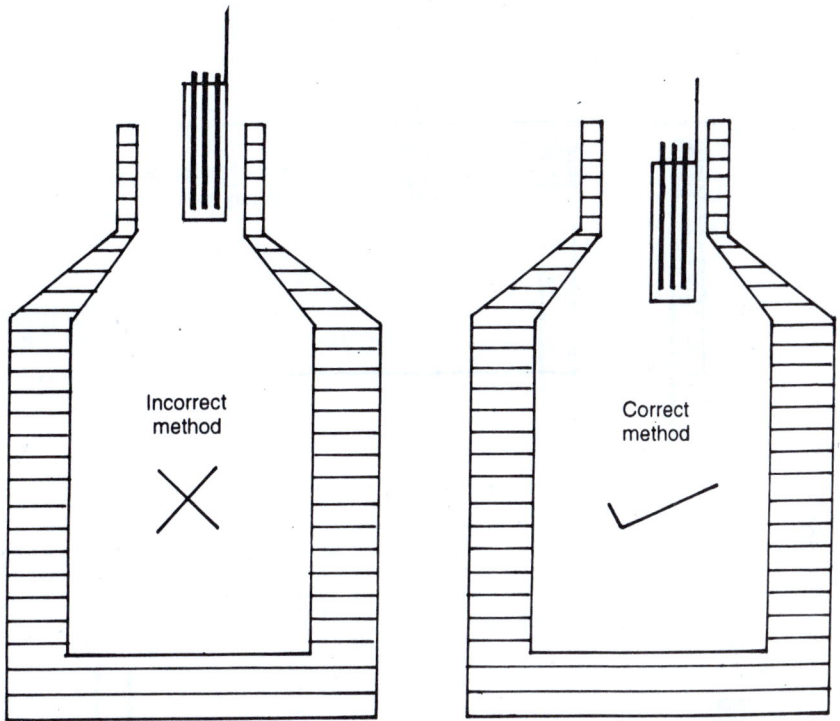

Fig. 18.2. Taking out straw(s) from liquid nitrogen container.

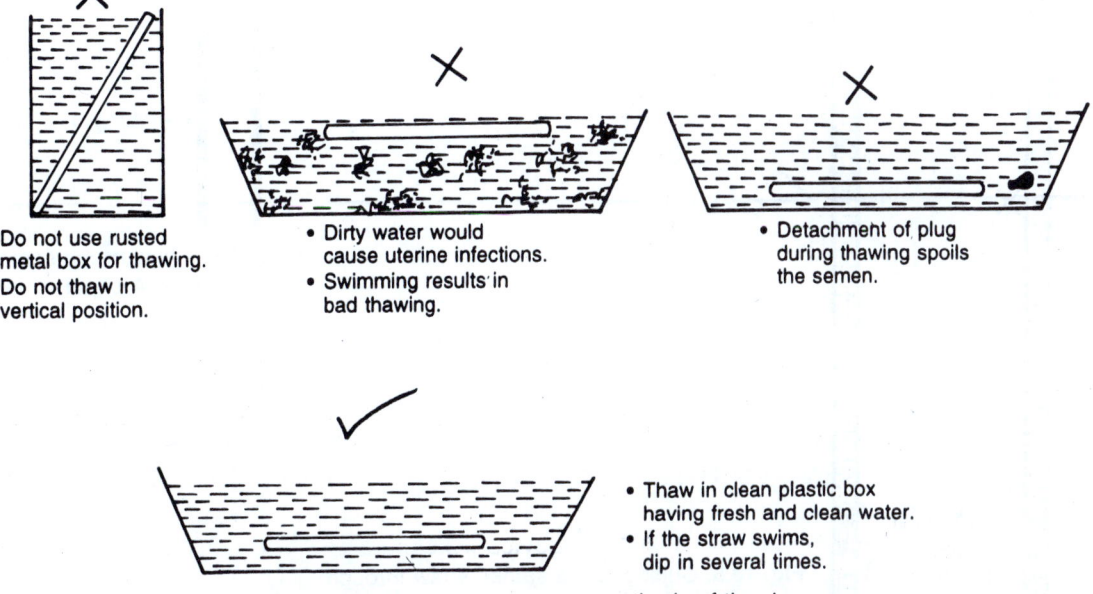

Do not use rusted
metal box for thawing.
Do not thaw in
vertical position.

- Dirty water would
  cause uterine infections.
- Swimming results in
  bad thawing.

- Detachment of plug
  during thawing spoils
  the semen.

- Thaw in clean plastic box
  having fresh and clean water.
- If the straw swims,
  dip in several times.

Fig. 18.3. Incorrect and correct methods of thawing.

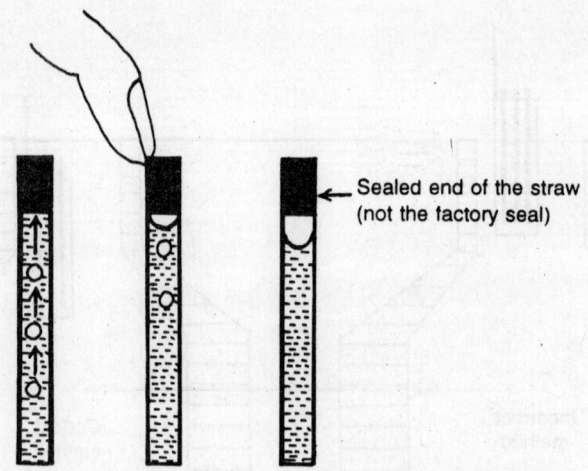

Sealed end of the straw (not the factory seal)

Fig. 18.4. Bringing up the air bubble just below single plug.

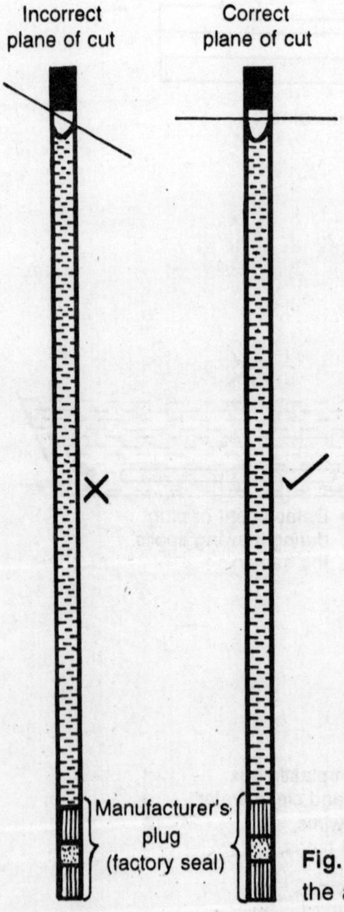

Incorrect plane of cut

Correct plane of cut

Manufacturer's plug (factory seal)

Fig. 18.5. Cutting of the semen straw through the air bubble to remove the seal plug.

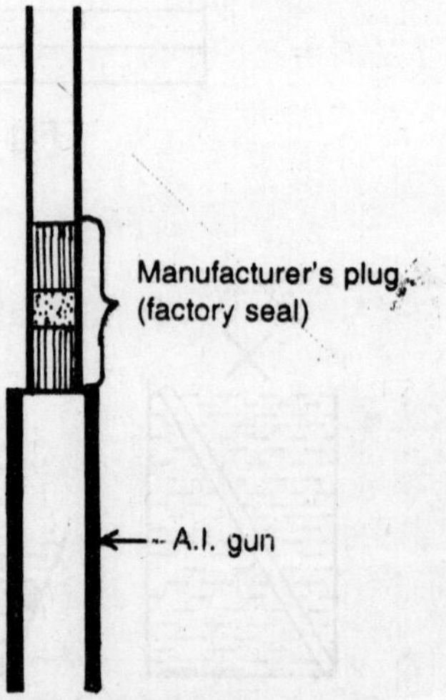

Manufacturer's plug (factory seal)

A.I. gun

Fig. 18.6. Fitting of the semen straw in to the A.I. gun.

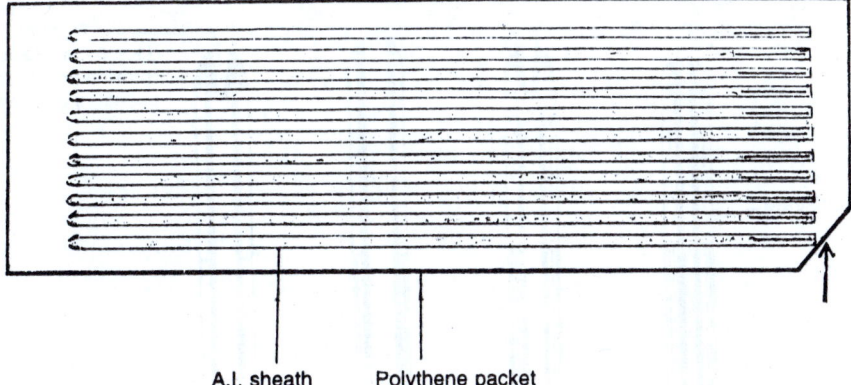

A.I. sheath   Polythene packet

Fig. 18.7. Polythene packet containing A.I. sheaths (↑ indicates cutting side towards the cut end of the sheaths).

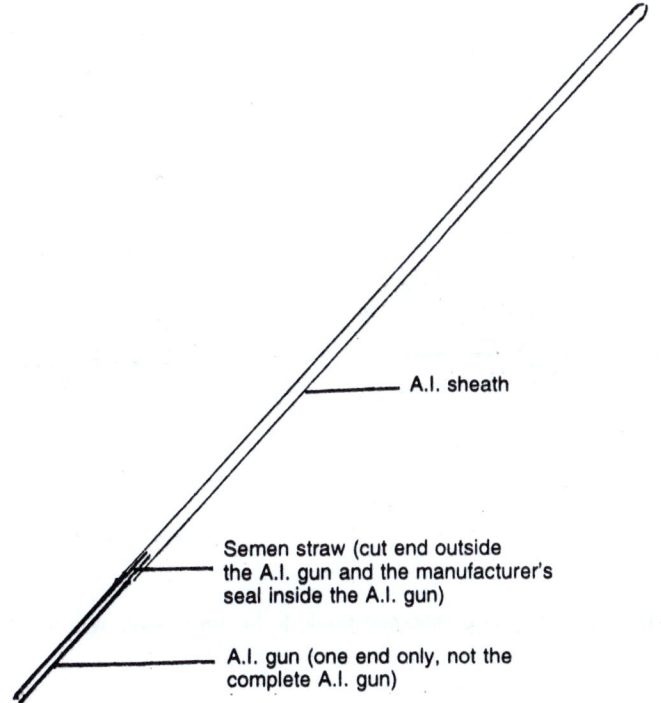

A.I. sheath

Semen straw (cut end outside the A.I. gun and the manufacturer's seal inside the A.I. gun)

A.I. gun (one end only, not the complete A.I. gun)

Fig. 18.8. Putting the sheath over A.I. gun loaded with semen straw.

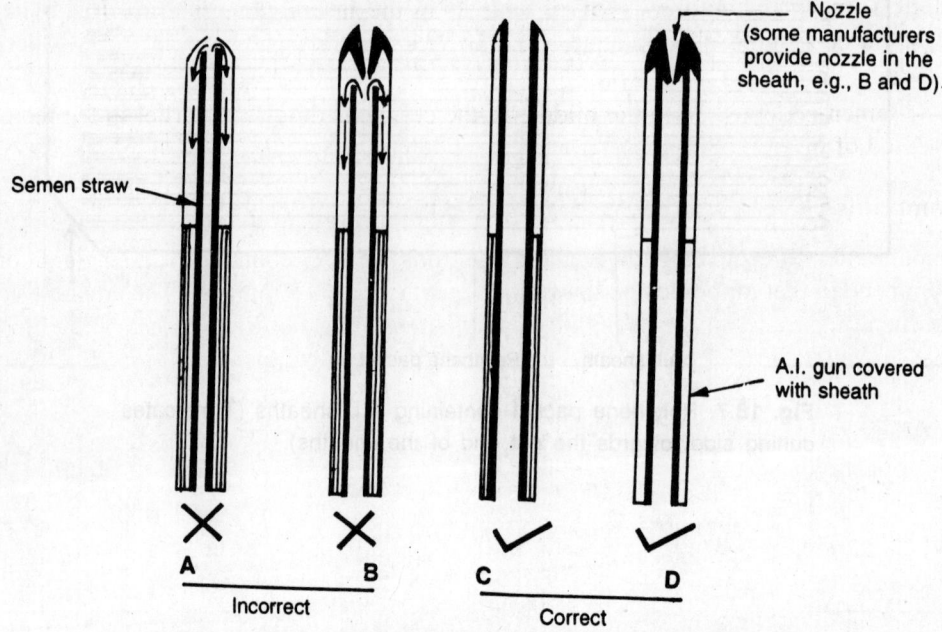

Fig. 18.9. Fixing of the cut end of the semen straw to the top of the sheath.

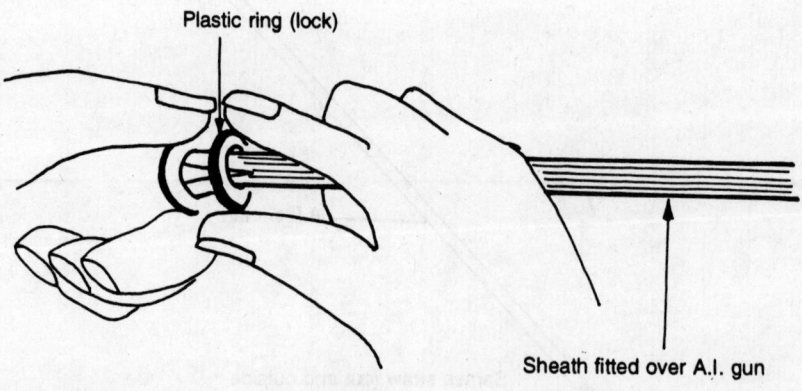

Fig. 18.10. Tightening of plastic ring (lock) to fix the sheath over the A.I. gun.

Note : Some manufacturers provide adapter in the inseminating sheath. If provided, the straw should be secured in the adapter (Fig. 18.9).

11. The semen is deposited in the middle of the cervix as described earlier in the recto-vaginal method of insemination.

Using ampoules

The ampoule after careful selection is taken out from the LN_2 container. Under field conditions, it is recommended that ampoules be thawed in ice water for 6-7 minutes. The ampoules are dried with absorbent material and are cut. The semen is drawn in a sterilized catheter fitted to a plastic or glass syringe with rubber connector. A.I. is done by recto-vaginal method as described earlier.

Chapter 19

Planning and Organization of Semen Collection and Artificial Insemination Centre

SEMEN COLLECTION CENTRE (BULL CENTRE)

The semen collection centre is itself a quite big concern where pedigreed bulls are kept in scientific manner in order to collect good quality semen. The semen collection centre should have space and facilities for day to day operations. Following are the essential requirements of the bull centre.

1. Bull paddocks
2. Semen collection shed
3. Laboratory for preliminary semen evaluation
4. Store for feed and fodder
5. Segregation ward for sick animals
6. Protected open area for exercise with facility of bull exerciser
7. Residential quarters for attendants

Bull Paddocks

Location

1. The semen collection centre should not be built in low lying area, where rain water, when accumulated is not drained out.
2. It should be located at a place where other personnels and animals may not have free access.
3. It should be located at a place well connected to places of semen distribution by all sorts of transports conveniently.
4. It should be located at a place having least disturbances.

Housing

The housing of individual bull in loose box with attached run is always preferred. For economy purpose the bulls may be tied in a single row in which each bull is separated by strong iron railing. Such an arrangement makes the feeding and watering of the bulls easy. But this arrangement has disadvantages too. The bulls remain in close contact to each other and whenever there is an outbreak of diseases, all bulls fall sick. The paddocks should be in a north-west to south-east direction in order to protect bulls from severe sun light and cold winds. The bull house should have an area of 16' × 16' with an open yard measuring 16' × 20'. The open air yard provide an opportunity to bull for natural exercise and also an exposure to sun. The room should have enough height. The ceiling height should be 10'-12'. The room should have enough light and ventilation. There should be a gap of 3'-4' between the roof and the ventilator. The roof should be such that could be easily cleaned. The paddocks should have a strong wall of at least 6' height to avoid undue excitement from neighbouring bulls. Such a height would also prevent the bulls from jumping outside the paddock. The floor should be non-slippery. The box stall and the paddock should have sufficient slope and drainage sysem. All corners of the house should be well rounded for better cleaning and disinfection. The feeding troughs should have semicircular shape so that the feed may fall back in the feeding trough and spoilage of the feed is minimized. The door should be wide and strong enough. The gate at the open pen should also be strong and at sufficient height. During summer buffalo bulls require comparatively cool house.

Semen Collection Shed

The semen collection shed should be at a convenient distance from the bull house to have full control on bulls. A short distance also helps in calling the bulls by their names. The semen collection shed should be comfortable to the bull. It should be free from direct sun-light and dust. Provision should be made for protection against cold and hot winds and also from showers of rain. The semen collection shed should have enough space. An area of 25' × 30' would be sufficient to install two crates(one for cattle bull and other for buffalo bull). Th crates should be strong enough and should be burried deep enough under the ground to prevent their dislocation. The crates should be made preferably of galvanized iron pipe. The crates should have wooden platform on either arm especially for buffalo bulls. The crates should have arrangements for fastening the neck of dummy. There should be provision also for fastening the rope leading the nose ring to avoid bull's escape. The semen collection shed should be a place of least disturbances. Adjacent to the crate, there should be strong guard railing of suitable height and the attendant leading the bull should always position himself across the guard rail so that he remains well protected. The floor of semen collection shed should be spread with thick layer of sand or soil and water should be sprinkled on it before semen collection. The site of collection should not be crowded with unwanted persons especially unfamiliar to the bulls.

Laboratory for preliminary semen evaluation

The semen, after collection should be examined as early as possible and hence the semen evaluation laboratory should be just near to the semen collection shed. A longer run may deteriorate semen quality. There should be, as far as possible, minimum entry of persons in the lab. The lab should have sliding glass window through which only the tube containing semen be passed in the lab and not the whole semen collection assembly. The sliding glass window should be opened only during passing the semen tube and should be closed immediately thereafter. The semen tube should be immediately placed in a water bath at 35-37°C. The semen collection lab should be clean, hygienic and dust free. It should have desirable electrical fittings with desirable light and points for electric connections in different equipment. There should be good supply of water together with wash basin. There should be good working bench and revolving stainless stools. The lab should have facility for ultra-violet radiation for sterilization. The inside temperature of the lab should be comofortable (around 30°C). There should be almirahs in the lab or another room attached to the lab for putting registers, sterilized glasswares and accessories of common use. There should be following materials/equipment in the lab.

1. Microscope attached with warm stage facility
2. Refrigerator
3. Water bath
4. Instrument cabinet for storing sterilized equipments
5. Absorbent cotton
6. Enamelled jugs and buckets
7. Test tube stands, measuring cylinders, beakers, flasks, test tubes (both ordinary and graduated)
8. Pipettes
9. Slides and cover slips
10. Polythene wash bottles
11. Spirit lamp
12. Aluminum foil
13. Eosin-Nigrosin stain
14. Waste basket
15. Electric heater
16. Extra electric plugs (5 and 15 amperes)
17. Kerosene oil stove
18. Minor instruments set (having screw driver, electric current tester etc.)
19. Artificial vagina
20. A.V. stand

Store for feed and fodder

The bull paddocks should have store for feed and fodder. Even if there is regular supply of fodder from outside, such stores would serve a useful purpose during emergencies when fodder supply is interrupted. The store should be such where fodder is not destroyed due to water or moisture. The fodder store should have wide door. The concentrate ration should be put in bags over wooden planks at least 6″ above the ground so as to save it from ground moisture. It should also be protected from rats etc.

Segregation ward for sick animals

The sick bulls should be placed in segregation wards. This would not only check the spread of disease to other bulls but would help also to pay attention to sick bulls. Segregation wards should be clean, dry, hygienic and comfortable to the animal and should have sufficient ventilation and light.

Protected open area for exercise with facility of "bull exerciser"

The bulls which are not sick should be given exercise daily. As it is not safe to carry the bulls to public roads, bull exerciser is very convenient for imparting exercise to bulls. It is better that a routine chart for the exercise of bulls is followed regularly. Under adverse weather conditions the exercise may be avoided or the timings may be changed. A walk of about 1-1.5 km daily is sufficient for bulls.

Residential quarters for attendants

In the bull shed any mishappening may occur at any time and if the bulls are not attended promptly during emergencies, it may become fatal. Hence, it is important that the bulls are kept in constant vigil. Therefore, the residential quarter of the attendant should not be far away from the bull shed. The residential quarters should be located at a place from where the bulls are easily watched and emergency situations are handled promptly.

INSEMINATION SHED

The insemination shed should be located at a place where animals may easily come for A.I. The A.I. shed should have roof for protection against rain and hot sun. The A.I. shed should have crate where animals can be fastened securely. The size of animals varies considerably and hence it is better that the A.I. shed should have crates of different sizes. There should be good supply of water and well drainage system on floor. The distance of A.I. shed from the semen laboratory should be convenient, short and approachable.

Chapter 20

Selection, Care, Training and Management of Bulls

It is a common saying that "A bull is half of the herd". The cows/buffaloes are receptive to males on estrum but the mature bulls are active to any estrous cow/buffalo at any time. The semen of cattle and buffalo bulls is collected artificially in a regular way for its maximum utilization through A.I. As such regular care of bulls is always essential to maintain them sound, both physically and reproductively. A regular calendar of operations for different managemental activities like feeding, watering, bathing, grooming, brushing, exercising, semen collection, paddock cleaning, health checkup, vaccination and testing for diseases like tuberculosis, Johne's disease etc. should be prepared in advance and should be strictly adhered to.

SELECTION OF BULLS

It is better to select the bulls in their early age i.e. about a year or so. Early selection helps in their proper care, feeding and management and for their proper training. Early selection also helps the bull to become adjusted with the environment in which they have to live. Before selection, the bull calves should undergo a very critical andrological examination.

ATTENDANTS

Both the attendants and the bulls should be familiar to each other. Regular changing of attendants should avoided. In no case all the attendants should be changed in one time. The persons engaged for feeding, watering, grooming, brushing, leading and exercise should be familiar to the bulls.

REGULAR HEALTH CHECKING

The breeding bulls should be checked daily. Any deviation e.g. poor feed intake, depression, uneasiness, fever, diarrhoea, constipation, cold, cough and bull's behaviour etc. should be noted cautiously. The whole body should be inspected thoroughly. The cause of disease should be investigated and treatment should be given promptly. Bulls suffering from infectious or contagious diseases should be immediately segregated from other bulls and put in segregation box. All health records of the bulls should be maintained.

EXERCISE

The bulls which are not sick should be given exercise daily. Exercise keeps their body tone fit and keeps them active. Morning exercise is better. If for some reason or the other the morning exercise is not possible, the bulls may be given exercise in the afternoon hours. Too extreme weathers are not suited for exercise. Bull exerciser is a very convenient tool for giving exercise to the bulls. Under no circumstances, the bulls should be taken to public roads for exercise. In the absence of the bull exerciser, the bulls may be given exercise in open but protected field. Buffalo bulls are difficult to harness in the bull exerciser. It is not safe too. The bulls have tendency to fight which may be fatal to bulls as well as to attendants and therefore loose handling of the bulls should always be avoided. Heavy and sudden exercise should always be avoided. It is better that regular chart of exercise to the bulls is followed. A total of about 1 km. walk on semen collection days and 2 km walk on days when the bulls are not utilized for semen collection is considered optimum for their exercise.

RESTRAINING OF BULLS

The bull should never be left free without restraint. The nose rings greatly help in restraining the bulls. The nose rings should be of better quality. The attendants can control a bull with the help of a rope fastened to the nose ring. A hook of suitable size attached securely to a strong and long wooden handle (about 5'-6' long) is of help in separating fighting bulls. Nose strings are also used across the nasal septum to have control on bull. Nylon ropes are found better compared to ropes made of cotton thread. Nylon ropes are more strong and more durable. Bulls should not be kept so loose that they may come close to each other and fight.

CLEANING, GROOMING AND BRUSHING

Daily cleaning operations on bull are advantageous to bull's health and these are beneficial to the attendants too looking after the bulls. Bulls, by nature are aggressive and daily handling of bulls by way of their cleaning, grooming, brushing, feeding and watering etc. make them to remain under control. The bulls should be given bath with fresh water daily as far as possible. Bathing may be stopped only occasionally under extremely cold weather conditions and in that case also their sheaths should be thoroughly washed. The grooming and brushing should be done daily. Grooming and brushing not only cleans the bull, but also help in better cutaneous circulation and in maintaining friendly relation with the bull. While cleaning, washing or grooming, the bull should be inspected for ectoparasites and harmful lesions. The area in between fore legs, between thighs, inguinal region, base of the tail and testicles should be washed carefully. Interdigital space should be thoroughly checked daily for the presence of any kind of lesions or foreign particle fastened. The preputial hairs should be clipped/shaved periodically. The buffalao bulls have affinity for wallowing and they enjoy 3-4 baths daily during summer months. Buffalo bulls may be shaved occasionally to keep them clean. Crows and other birds are seen coming and sitting on bull's back. These birds generally come and pick parasites and debris on their humps, base of the horn or near tail head. If there are wounds on the body, pricking by birds may cause further damage. Daily cleaning, grooming and brushing would keep the animal clean and healthy and would thus prevent pricking by crows and other birds. Bulls should be well cleaned and properly dried before they are taken for semen collection.

VACCINATION AND TESTING OF DISEASES

The bulls should be prevented against diseases using prophylactic vaccines like Foot and Mouth disease, Rinderpest, Hemorrhagic septicemia, Black-quarter and Anthrax etc. It is always better that a vaccination schedule be planned in advance and this should be strictly adhered. The venereal or semen borne diseases have a special concern in the examination of the bulls for their breeding soundness. All records of vaccination should be properly maintained. The bulls should also be tested periodically against Brucellosis, Campylobacteriosis, Trichomoniasis, Tuberculosis, Leptospirosis and Johne's disease (Paratuberculosis). Faecal examination and deworming should be adopted as a routine practice in bulls.

TRAINING TO YOUNGER BULLS

The training to the young bulls for donating semen be stared in their young age. It is better to impart training in the morning hours when their stomach is light and the bulls are active. In summer, the training may be started early morning and in winter in between 8-9 a.m. The bulls should be prepared clean as for routine semen collection. The bulls may be made familiar to the site of semen collection in advance. They respond well in familiar environment. It is always helpful, if the bulls are familiar to the dummy. The bulls may be allowed to ride over first on anestrous females but these females should be well clean and free from any disease and then on male dummy. The anestrous female or male dummy should be kept well secured in the crate and in no way these be allowed to kick or hurt the bulls. The furious dummy would spoil the training of the young bulls. The younger and untrained bulls are timid in nature and if are hurt would not donate semen easily. The size of anestrous female or male dummy should be according to the size of the bull. The younger bulls may be allowed to observe from distance, the process of semen donation by other bulls. When the younger bulls start nuzzling and licking of vulva these may be allowed to ride over dummy, but by this time the semen collector should be perfectly ready. During riding and ejaculation, kind words and whistling greatly stimulate the process. The operator should have patience as the process may take hours. Some bulls have affinity for certain dummies or for certain colours and such things if noted, should be harnessed to their maximum for semen collection. Proper temperature and pressure of the A.V. is always important. The temperature of other A.V. should be kept around 41°C. When the bulls start donating semen, the semen should be collected daily for 3-4 days and then a regular semen collection schedule should be followed.

FEEDING OF BULLS

The kind of feeds and fodder available would change from place to place and from season to season. The feeding schedule should be worked out depending upon its availability and the requirements by the bull. The bull grows up to the age of about 5 years and during this period the ration provided should be growth promoting and should contain enough protein. Thereafter the ration would depend upon the maintenance requirements as well as production requirements depending upon the frequency of semen ejaculation. Green fodder is an essential requirement of bulls. In the absence of green fodder vitamin-A should be supplemented in the diet. The concentrate ration should contain enough amount of protein, carbohydrates and mineral mixture. Reasonable quantity of DCP and TDN should be given to the bulls. If good quality of feed is fed to the bulls, 2 to 3 kg of concentrate ration would be sufficient to keep the bull in desired condition depending upon their live weight and frequency of service. The requirements of DCP, TDN, carotene, calcium and phosphorus required for growing and adult bulls are given in Tables 20.1 and 20.2.

Table 20.1. Nutrients requirement for Growing Bull Calves

Live weight (kg)	DCP (kg)	TDN (kg)	Carotene (mg)	Calcium (gm)	Phosphorus (gm)
100	0.28	1.9	11	13	10
150	0.35	2.6	16	13	12
200	0.40	3.0	21	13	12
300	0.45	4.0	32	13	12
400	0.48	5.0	40	12	12

Table 20.2. Nutrients Requirement for Bulls in Service

Live weight (kg)	DCP (kg)	TDN (kg)	Carotene (mg)	Calcium (gm)	Phosphorus (gm)
400	0.38	3.6	45	9	9
500	0.45	4.5	55	11	11
600	0.53	5.4	66	13	13

From : Nutritive Values of Indian Cattle Feeds and the Feeding of Animals by K.C. Sen, S.N. Ray and S.K. Ranjan (ICAR).

VICES IN BULLS

Vices may develop in bulls due to improper and abusive handling, long confinement in dark, lack of exercise, abnormal surroundings and associations provided with other females and castrated males. Behavioural disorders may affect copulatory efficiency.

Masturbation or Onanism

It is observed in males of all the species. This vice has no significant effect on fertility or libido but in such bulls, semen cannot be obtained with certainty. Irregularity of semen collection may be a factor for developing this vice. This vice would decline by regular and frequent use of the bull for semen collection. Hygiene and regular exercise in- and outside the paddock would also help to avoid masturbation.

Viciousness

It is the vice because of confinement and abusive treatment to the bull like teasing, irritating and malhandling. The wicked bull, if chronic, is very difficult to manage. Proper handling of the bull from young age and daily washing, cleaning, grooming, brushing and exercise together with kindness to the bull help in overcoming the vicious nature of the bull.

Slowness in breeding (sluggish breeders)

Slowness in breeding may be associated with low endocrine status, however, this may also occur due to improper and abusive handling or other painful experiences during past ejaculations.

Lack of sexual desire

Lack of sexual desire is primarily due to low endocrine status and is determined genetically but the environmental factors also play an important role in modifying it, e.g. poor or faulty feeding, systemic diseases, old age and faulty management practices.

Chapter 21

Recording Systems for Andrology and A.I.

Systematic recording of all the reproductive parameters and reproductive events, weather in semen producing unit or in any A.I. centre can never be underestimated. All the information regarding reproductive parameters and events be recorded in a easy and systematic way so that relevant information may be traced easily. The bull produces many off-springs. The efficiency changes from bull to bull. The performance of the bull should always be evaluated for their economic characters so as to select better bulls and further the bulls should be evaluated for economic characteristics in the progeny in their earliest possible life time. The fertility also differs from bull to bull. Females also do not breed with similar rate. For better economics early conversion of heifers into cows, minimum possible intercalving period and least occurrence of reproductive problem are essential. The best females should be allowed to remain in the herd and the defaulters or problem breeders should be culled. The working efficiency also differs from inseminator to inseminator. A lot of expenditure is done on the salary of the inseminator. Better conception rate would certainly be economical. Hence it is also important that the work carried out by different inseminators should be evaluated. In nut shell following information would be essential.

1. Data from different bulls regarding semen collection, semen evaluation, semen preservation and semen distribution to various A.I. centres.
2. Fertility results from different bulls.
3. Records to reproductive performance of the females together with abnormalities, if any.
4. Data regarding the work carried out by different inseminators.

There cannot be a very rigid system for recording. The recording may differ from place to place and from organization to organization. However, for the recording of above information, the following registers/individual cards should be maintained.

1. Semen collection register
2. Bull performance register
3. Register/individual cards for reproduction records of individual females
4. Insemination register

(Refer Proforma given in Exercises 16, 17, 18 and 19.)

Chapter 22

Cleaning and Sterilization of A.I. Equipment and Their Upkeep

CLEANING

Immediately after use all the A.I. equipment should be washed thoroughly with water. Semen/egg yolk etc. when remain adhered in the capillary of the A.I. catheter or remain sticked to other glassware, get dry after some time and then it becomes difficult to clean the glasswares. All A.I. catheters should be washed immediately after use by putting them under tap so that the semen remaining in A.I. catheters is washed with the force of water. The glassware may then be put in chromic acid solution for overnight dip. This would help removing cloudiness from glassware. The application of corrosive substances on rubber-wares should be avoided. Corrosive substances reduce the life of rubber articles. The articles are then washed with lukewarm soap solution using brush to make the articles grease free. The equipment are now washed thoroughly, several times, under tap water and are put inverted in a clean tray. Finally the articles are rinsed with distilled water to avoid deposits of any salt and they appear clean on drying. The artificial vagina may be thoroughly cleaned using lukewarm detergent solution and brush. There is no need of separating inner rubber lining from the hard rubber cylinder. The A.V. should then be washed thoroughly with water. The laboratories should be cleaned preferably with vacuum cleaner.

STERILIZATION

Unsterilized A.I. equipment may become a potential source of infection. The infection may spread to the female genital tract and also the microorganisms and their products may injure the spermatozoa and may result in rapid decline in the quality of the stored spermatozoa. All sorts of equipment which are used for semen collection, preparation of buffers, semen dilution, semen storage and during artificial insemination must be infection free. Sterilization means either physical or chemical treatments to eliminate all possible microbes from the equipment. Sterilization of all the equipment used in various processes of semen collection, buffer preparation, semen dilution, semen handling and during artificial insemination should be a regular practice without any negligence.

Dry Heat Sterilization

Dry heat sterilization is generally preferred for glass wares and metallic wares. The dry heat sterilization process is easy and rapid and all the organisms are susceptible to dry heat sterilization. The heat penetrates deeply in clumps and reaches surfaces that might remain protected by disinfectants. The pathogenic bacteria, viruses and fungi are killed within few minutes at 50-70°C and the spores of various pathogens are killed at 100°C. It is a common practice to sterilize all glassware and metallic wares in hot air oven at 180-200°C for 1 hr.

The opening (mouth) of the properly cleaned and washed glassware and metallic wares should be closed with paper. The articles which do not have opening or the articles of which sterilization of outer surface is important during use (e.g. A.I. catheters) should be wrapped in paper.

Autoclaving

Sterilization by autoclaving is a very popular method. The rapid action of sterilization by autoclaving is largely due to latent heat of water vapor (540 cal/gm). For using autoclave, it is important to keep in mind that flowing steam be allowed to displace the air before closing the valve. In the steam mixed with air, the temperature would be less and moreover heating would be uneven since the air would tend to remain at the bottom of the chamber. All rubber articles and artificial vagina may be autoclaved at 10 1b (4 kg) pressure at 115.6°C for 20 minutes. Higher pressure would spoil and change the shape of such articles. Other articles including buffer solutions and Vaseline may be autoclaved at 17 1b (7 kg) pressure at 121°C for 15-20 minutes. The buffers may also be autoclaved. Solutions containing sugars should not be autoclaved. Autoclaving destroys sugars. All vessels to be sterilized by autoclaving should be either loosely plugged or capped and should not be filled completely, if containing any solution, in order to permit free passage of dissolved air during heating and free heating of the superheated liquid when the steam pressure is lowered. Immediately after autoclaving the articles (except solutions) should be kept in oven at around 40°C for drying. Sterilized articles must be stored in air-tight cabinets. Hot air oven or incubators at 40°C may also be used as storage cabinets The buffer solutions after autoclaving, should be cooled down to room temperature and should be stored in refrigerator for use.

Ultraviolet Radiation

The energy of the ultraviolet radiation is absorbed by the molecules of the appropriate structure. The absorbing molecule is activated resulting in either increased interatomic vibration or excitation of electron to higher energy levels. There may be rupture of bonds, formation of new bonds and the same changes may occur in adjacent molecules because of transfer of energy to these molecules. The ultraviolet absorption of bacteria is due chiefly by purines and pyrimidines of nucleic acids and less to aromatic rings of tryptophan, tyrosine, and phenylalanine of proteins. The absorption of ultraviolet radiation by nucleic acid and protein causes lethal effect. The effectiveness of ultraviolet radiation is well proved and sterilization of semen processing lab may be done using inexpensive, low pressure mercury-vapor lamps.

Gaseous Sterilization (Ethylene Oxide)

Ethylene oxide is an effective sterilizing agent at low temperature with good penetrating power under desirable standards. Ethylene oxide is a gas at room temperature and vapourises at 10.8°C. Ethylene oxide is a highly water soluble gas and is used for gaseous disinfection of dry surfaces.

However, its use is more expensive and presents more hazard of residual toxicity. The potential hazard of mutagenicity and carcinogenicity for human beings deserves thorough investigations since ethylene oxide has been shown to cause mutagenicity of bacteria and plant seeds. Ethylene oxide is used to sterilize heat labile and moisture sensitive objects like rubber, electronic equipment and plastic wares. Well cleaned and washed plastic wares are put in polythene bags. The polythene bags are sealed and the sealed bags are sterilized in Ethylene oxide chamber. Freoxide is a mixture of Ethylene oxide (12%) and Freon (88%) and is also used for gas sterilization.

EQUIPMENT OF AN A.I. UNIT USING FROZEN SEMEN AND ITS UPKEEP

Standard Items

1. Liquid nitrogen container(s) with frozen semen
2. Dip stick for measuring the level of liquid nitrogen
3. A.I. gun appropriate to the type of frozen semen straw (midi/mini)
4. Plastic sheaths in sufficient number appropriate to the type of frozen semen straw in intact polythene bag
5. Semen straw holding forceps
6. Thawing box
7. Clean absorbent cotton/clean cloth for absorbing moisture from thawed semen straw
8. Clean and sharp scissors for cutting the sealed end of the straw
9. A clean and hygienic tray for carrying A.I. gun, sheaths, scissors and straw holding forceps etc.
10. Soap and clean towel
11. Centigrade thermometer for checking temperature of the thaw bath
12. Enamelled jug and bucket for water
13. Register/Cards for records regarding artificial inseminations done

Liquid Nitrogen Container, its Construction and Precautions in Handling

Liquid nitrogen containers are not so tough as they appear by their secured external appearance. In fact, liquid nitrogen containers are delicate by construction and because of mishandling due to lack of knowledge about its internal construction, premature destruction of liquid nitrogen containers is very common. Liquid nitrogen containers are very costly and their premature destruction should always be avoided. A high quality and intact liquid nitrogen container would lead to least possible evaporation of the liquid nitrogen. The liquid nitrogen container is double layered vessel (Fig. 22.1). The inner chamber is suspended in the outer chamber through neck tube which is non-metal and a bad conductor of heat. This structure (neck tube) prevents transfer of heat from outside to the inner chamber and thus rapid evaporation of the liquid nitrogen is prevented. The neck tube is a weaker structure compared to metallic parts. The addition of liquid nitrogen in the liquid nitrogen containers increases considerably the weight load that the neck tube must support. Sudden moves and jerks vibrate the inner chamber. Thus side to side movement of the inner chamber puts considerable stress on neck tube which is non-metal and delicate and very often leads to mechanical damage. The wall of the inner chamber is coated with high quality insulating material. High quality insulating material is also filled in between the outer and inner chambers. Vacuum is created in between the inner and the outer chambers. In the absence of the vacuum the liquid nitrogen would

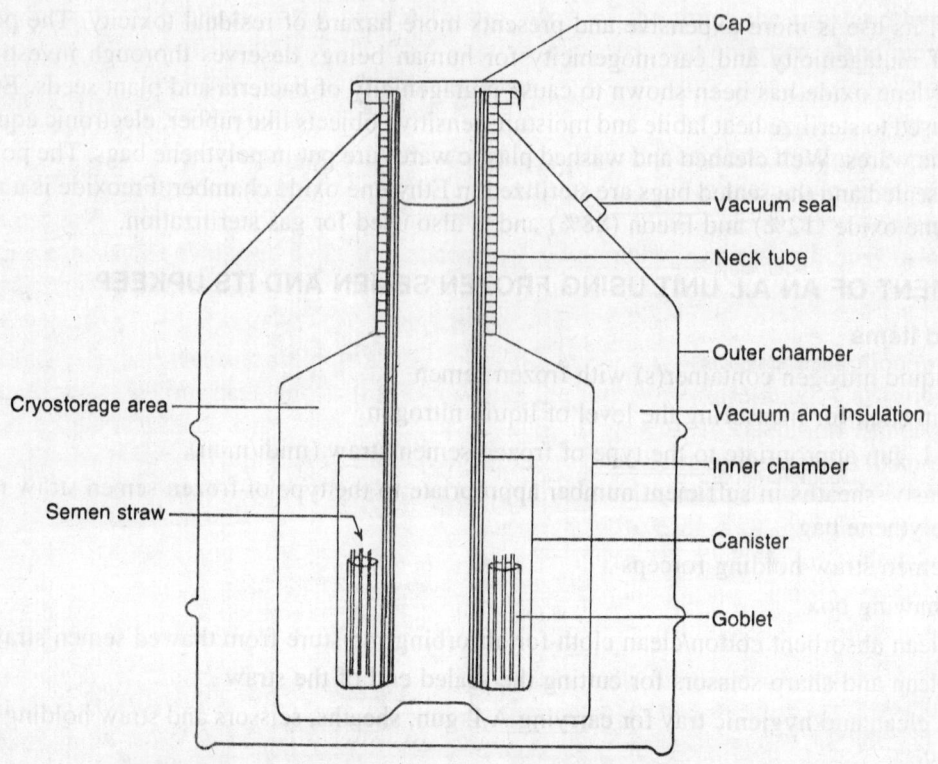

Fig. 22.1. Liquid nitrogen container showing inner construction.

boil and there would be rapid loss of liquid nitrogen from the inner chamber. A highly visible frost at the top of the liquid nitrogen container is indicative of rapid evaporation of the liquid nitrogen.

Precautions

1. Liquid nitrogen containers should be kept in a cold place. Exposure to direct sun light and hot air should be avoided.
2. The room for storing liquid nitrogen containers (filled with liquid nitrogen) should be well ventilated.
3. Avoid direct contact of liquid nitrogen containers with hard floor. Use rubber/jute mats.
4. Avoid moisture on floor.
5. Avoid injuries, drilling, puncturing and scrapping.
6. Do not play with vacuum knob.
7. Never roll the liquid nitrogen containers. Pull or push with friction on floor should always be avoided. Do not swing the liquid nitrogen containers. Always avoid abrupt contact with door frames, and other fixed objects.
8. Use trolley in the transportation of the liquid nitrogen containers.
9. Do not put liquid nitrogen containers one over other.
10. Never change lid from other containers.
11. Always keep the lid loaded over the container (except during putting in or taking out frozen semen).

12. Always use the lid in straight upright position while putting it on or off the liquid nitrogen containers.

13. Do not interchange canisters from other liquid nitrogen containers. The canisters are specific to the design of the liquid nitrogen containers and reach to the bottom of the inner chamber. This position helps to keep the frozen semen dipped in liquid nitrogen. If the canister's size is not appropriate, it would either not fit well or would not reach to the bottom of the inner chamber of the liquid nitrogen container.

14. Fill the liquid nitrogen slowly.

15. Make regular checks of the liquid nitrogen in the container. Any increase in the expected evaporation rate should be taken seriously.

16. Do not put undesired material in the liquid nitrogen containers.

Dip Stick for Measuring the Level of Liquid Nitrogen in the Container

Checks regarding the level of liquid nitrogen in the cryocan are made by dipping a ruler in the cryocan. The dip stick (Fig. 22.2) should strike the bottom of the cryocan and should remain in

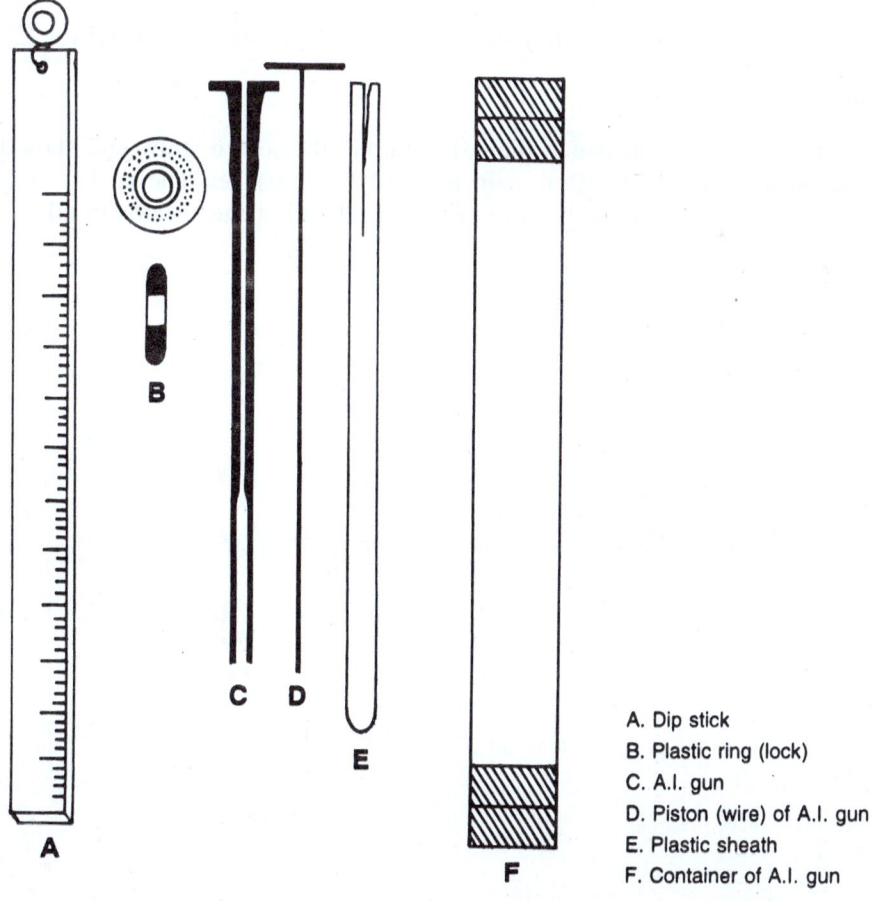

A. Dip stick
B. Plastic ring (lock)
C. A.I. gun
D. Piston (wire) of A.I. gun
E. Plastic sheath
F. Container of A.I. gun

Fig. 22.2. Some items required in A.I. with frozen semen straws.

the tank for about 10 seconds. Once the dip stick is removed from the liquid nitrogen container and is waved in air, frost is formed on it, in just few seconds. The frost indicates the level of the liquid nitrogen in the liquid nitrogen container. Black coloured dip stick is preferred, since it provides a good contrast between white frost and black coloured dip stick.

Precautions

1. Unnecessary and frequent measuring of the liquid nitrogen level should be avoided. It leads to unnecessary evaporation of liquid nitrogen.
2. Dip stick should not be kept loose, otherwise it may break. It should be hanged through wall.

A.I. Gun

The A.I. gun (Fig. 22.2) should match the straw of frozen semen and should always be kept clean and hygienic.

Precautions

1. Care should be taken to avoid bending of A.I. gun and piston wire.
2. It should be clean and hygienic.
3. For further protection, A.I. gun may be kept in plastic/perpex container (Fig. 22.2).

Plastic Sheaths

Plastic sheaths (Fig. 22.2) should match the A.I. gun and the semen straw and should never be kept loose. The sheaths should always remain in a polythene packet. The packet of the sheaths should be given a small cut towards the side of the broad end of the sheaths to take out sheaths for use.

EXERCISE 1

Date . . . .

HISTORY OF THE BULL FOR BREEDING SOUNDNESS

Name/No. of the bull . . . . Date of birth/Age . . . .

Owner's name & address . . . .

. . . .

Permanent markings . . . .

. . . .

. . . .

1. **Breed** . . . .
2. **Genetic group** . . . .
3. **Percentage of exotic blood** . . . .
4. **Dam's yield** . . . .
5. **Grand dam's yield** . . . .
6. **Yield of progeny** (if known) . . . .
7. **Fertility** (if known) . . . .
8. **Abnormalities in females after service**
   (a) Abnormal discharge . . . .
   (b) Delayed return of estrum . . . .
   (c) Abortion . . . .
   (d) Lethal/Semilethal/Undesired
       characteristics in the progeny . . . .
   (e) Others . . . .
9. **Surgical operations**
   (a) Hernia . . . .
   (b) Penile deviation . . . .
   (c) Others . . . .

10. **Vaccination history**

	Date	Vaccine & dose
(a) F.M.D.	. . . .	. . . .
(b) H.S.	. . . .	. . . .
(c) B.Q.	. . . .	. . . .
(d) R.P.	. . . .	. . . .
(e) Others	. . . .	. . . .

11. **Previous service behavior**
    (excellent/good/fair/poor)   . . . .

12. **Remarks**

13. **Precautions**

Signature of Student   Signature of Instructor

EXERCISE 2

Date . . . .

GENERAL EXAMINATION OF THE BULL
FOR BREEDING SOUNDNESS

Name/No. of the bull . . . . Date of birth/Age . . . .

Owner's name & address . . . .

. . . .

Permanent markings . . . .

. . . .

. . . .

1. **Physical condition**

   (a) Body weight . . . .

   (b) General condition
   (normal/obese/thin/emaciated) . . . .

   (c) Temperament (furious/masculine &
   somewhat aggressive/feminine and docile) . . . .

   (d) Activeness (alert/dull) . . . .

   (e) Response to external stimuli
   (e.g. with movement and sound) . . . .

   (f) Vision (normal/defective) . . . .

   (g) Shoulder built (massive and
   developed/reduced) . . . .

   (h) Hump (in zebu cattle bulls)
   [e.g. (i) massive/less developed;
   (ii) erect/leaning to one side] . . . .

   (i) Skin coat (smooth and shining/dull) . . . .

   (j) Any other finding . . . .

2. **Integument**

   (a) Hernia . . . .

   (b) Tumor . . . .

   (c) Any other finding . . . .

3. **Digestive system**
   (a) Prehension of food . . . .
   (b) Mastication of food . . . .
   (c) Swallowing of food . . . .
   (d) Posture during eating . . . .
   (e) Posture during defecation . . . .
   (f) Appetite . . . .
   (g) Rumination . . . .
   (h) Mucus membrane of the oral cavity . . . .
   (i) Tongue . . . .
   (j) Teeth . . . .
   (k) Feces
       (i) Colour . . . .
       (ii) Consistency . . . .
       (iii) Amount . . . .
       (iv) Smell . . . .
       (v) Mucus . . . .
       (vi) Blood . . . .
       (vii) Parasites . . . .
       (viii) Other findings . . . .
   (l) Other findings (if any) . . . .

4. **Urinary system**
   (a) Posture during urination . . . .
   (b) Frequency of urination . . . .
   (c) Pain during urination . . . .
   (d) Colour of urine . . . .
   (e) Amount of urine . . . .
   (f) Any other finding . . . .

5. **Circulatory system**
   (a) Pulse rate . . . .
   (b) Nature of pulse . . . .
   (c) Auscultation of heart . . . .
   (d) Percussion of heart . . . .
   (e) Any other finding . . . .

6. **Lymphatic system**

   Name of lymph gland(s)

   (a) Size . . . .
   (b) Pain reaction . . . .
   (c) Lobulations . . . .

(d) Consistency . . . .

(e) Temperature of the overlying skin . . . .

(f) Abscesses . . . .

(g) Any other finding . . . .

7. **Respiratory system**

(a) Respiration rate . . . .

(b) Regularity of respiration . . . .

(c) Depth of respiration . . . .

(d) Thoracic/abdominal respiration . . . .

(e) Pain during respiration . . . .

(f) Cough . . . .

(g) Nasal discharge . . . .

(h) Any other finding . . . .

8. **Neuromusculoskeletal and hooves (NMHS) system**

(a) Conformation of legs

(i) From back . . . .

(ii) From sides . . . .

(iii) Joints . . . .

(iv) Angles of joints . . . .

(v) Base of foot . . . .

(vi) Symmetry of hooves . . . .

(vii) Pain . . . .

(viii) Gait . . . .

(ix) Paralysis . . . .

(x) Weight bearing capacity . . . .

(xi) Any other finding . . . .

9. **Remarks**

10. **Precautions**

Signature of Student   Signature of Instructor

EXERCISE 3

Date . . . .

EXAMINATION OF BULL'S GENITALIA (EXTERNALIA AND INTERNALIA) FOR BREEDING SOUNDNESS

Name/No. of the bull . . . . Date of birth/Age . . . .
Owner's name & address . . . .
. . . .
Permanent markings . . . .
. . . .
. . . .

1. **Examination of externalia**

		Right testis	Left testis
(A)	Testes		
	(a) Shape	. . . .	. . . .
	(b) Length	. . . .	. . . .
	(c) Circumference	. . . .	. . . .
	(d) Adhesions with scrotum	. . . .	. . . .
	(e) Hypoplasia	. . . .	. . . .
	(f) Cryptorchidism	. . . .	. . . .
	(g) Any other finding	. . . .	. . . .
(B)	Scrotum		
	(a) Nature of scrotal wall	. . . .	. . . .
	(b) Presence of fat	. . . .	. . . .
	(c) Presence of Varicocele	. . . .	. . . .
	(d) Scrotal hernia	. . . .	. . . .
	(e) Twisting	. . . .	. . . .
	(f) Any other findings	. . . .	. . . .
(C)	Epididymis		
	(a) Abscess	. . . .	. . . .
	(b) Unusual enlargement	. . . .	. . . .
	(c) Atrophy	. . . .	. . . .
	(d) Hypertrophy	. . . .	. . . .

     (e) Pain on palpation   . . . .

     (f) Anatomical arrangement   . . . .

     (g) Any other finding   . . . .

(D) Penis

     (a) Development   . . . .

     (b) Inflammation   . . . .

     (c) Fracture   . . . .

     (d) Anatomical defect   . . . .

     (e) Deviation   . . . .

     (f) Adhesion   . . . .

     (g) Any other finding   . . . .

(E) Prepuce

     (a) Inflammation   . . . .

     (b) Abnormal discharge   . . . .

     (c) Presence of frenulum   . . . .

     (d) Eversion of prepuce   . . . .

     (e) Pendulous prepuce/sheath   . . . .

     (f) Any other finding   . . . .

2. Examination of internalia

(A) Ampullae

     (a) Ampullitis   . . . .

     (b) Hypoplasia   . . . .

     (c) Hyperplasia   . . . .

     (d) Pain on palpation   . . . .

     (e) Any other finding   . . . .

(B) Vesicular glands

     (a) Shape   . . . .

     (b) Lobulations   . . . .

     (c) Consistency   . . . .

     (d) Aplasia   . . . .

     (e) Hyperplasia   . . . .

     (f) Pain on palpation   . . . .

     (g) Any other finding   . . . .

3. Other related observations

(A) Libido   . . . .

(B) Thrust   . . . .

(C) Secondary sexual characteristics   . . . .

4. **Remarks**

5. **Precautions**

Signature of Student   **Signature of Instructor**

EXERCISE 4

Date . . . .

PREPARATION OF A.V. AND COLLECTION OF SEMEN

1. **Materials required**
    1. . . . .
    2. . . . .
    3. . . . .
    4. . . . .

    5. . . . .
    6. . . . .
    7. . . . .
    8. . . . .

2. **Different parts of A.V.**
    1. . . . .
    2. . . . .
    3. . . . .

    4. . . . .
    5. . . . .
    6. . . . .

3. **Assembling the artificial vagina**

4. **Pre-warming and warming of artificial vagina**

5. **Semen collection** (method)

6. **Quantity and quality of semen obtained**
   Appearance   . . . .
   Colour   . . . .
   Mass motility   . . . .
   Volume   . . . . ml
   Odour   . . . .
   Foreign bodies   . . . .

7. **Remarks**

8. **Precautions**

Signature of Student   Signature of Instructor

EXERCISE 5

Date . . . .

SEMEN EVALUATION

A. Sperm Concentration

1. **Materials required**

    1. . . . .   4. . . . .

    2. . . . .   5. . . . .

    3. . . . .   6. . . . .

2. **Preparation of diluting fluid**

3. **Steps** (method)

4. **Calculations**

5. **Result**

The sperm concentration in the given semen sample is .... /ml

6. **Precautions**

7. **Precautions**

Signature of Student   Signature of Instructor

EXERCISE 6

Date . . . .

SEMEN EVALUATION (Continued)

B. Live Spermatozoa (%)

  1. **Materials required**

      1. . . . .   4. . . . .

      2. . . . .   5. . . . .

      3. . . . .   6. . . . .

  2. **Preparation of eosin-nigrosin stain**

      What does eosin do?

      What does nigrosin do?

  3. **Method of slide preparation**

  4. **Counting of live/dead sperms**

5. **Results**
   1. Number of sperms counted ....
   2. Number of live sperms ....
   3. Live spermatozoa are .... %

   The semen .... may/may not be used.

6. **Remarks**

7. **Precautions**

Signature of Student   Signature of Instructor

EXERCISE 7

Date . . . .

SEMEN EVALUATION (Continued)

C. Sperm Abnormalities

The same slide prepared for the estimation of live spermatozoa is used for the estimation of sperm abnormalities.

1. **Counting of sperm abnormalities**

2. **Results**

    No. of sperm cells counted . . . .

	Abnormalities		
	Primary	Secondary	Total
Head	. . . .	. . . .	. . . .
Middle piece	. . . .	. . . .	. . . .
Tail	. . . .	. . . .	. . . .
		Grand total	

   Total sperm abnormalities = ... %

   The semen . . . . may/may not be used.

3. **Remarks**

4. **Precautions**

Signature of Student   Signature of Instructor

EXERCISE 8

Date . . . .

SEMEN EVALUATION (Continued)

D. Methylene Blue Reduction Test

  1. **Principle**

  2. **Materials required**

     1. . . . .   4. . . . .

     2. . . . .   5. . . . .

     3. . . . .   6. . . . .

  3. **Preparation of methylene blue solution**

  4. **Method**

5. Results

Time taken for the disappearance of blue colour (Decolouration of semen : Methylene blue suspension) = ... minutes

The sperm sample is of .... quality

(Excellent/average/poor)

6. Remarks

7. Precautions

Signature of Student   Signature of Instructor

EXERCISE 9

Date . . . .

PREPARATION OF DILUTOR AND DILUTION OF SEMEN

1. **Basic principles/functions of semen dilutors**
   1. . . . .
   2. . . . .
   3. . . . .
   4. . . . .
   5. . . . .

2. **Name of dilutor**

3. **Materials required**

   1.   5. . . . .
   2.   6. . . . .
   3.   7. . . . .
   4.   8. . . . .

4. **Composition of dilutor** (. . . . .)
   (Name of the dilutor)

5. **Extension of semen**
   Motility of spermatozoa . . . . %
   Sperm concentration . . . . millions/ml
   Calculations for semen dilution

Final dilution ratio = 1 :

(Semen : dilutor)

6. **Observations**

Motility of spermatozoa in diluted sample = ... %

7. **Remarks**

8. **Precautions**

Signature of Student   Signature of Instructor

EXERCISE 10

Date . . . .

PRESERVATION OF SEMEN AT AMBIENT AND REFRIGERATION TEMPERATURES

A. Name of the Dilutor

1. **Materials required**

   1. . . . .   5. . . . .
   2. . . . .   6. . . . .
   3. . . . .   7. . . . .
   4. . . . .   8. . . . .

2. **Composition of the dilutor**

3. **Extension of semen**

4. **Storage temperature** .... °C

5. **Observations**

   The sperm motility in .... dilutor after .... hrs. of preservation is
   .... %

6. **Remarks**

7. **Precautions**

Signature of Student   Signature of Instructor

EXERCISE 11

Date . . . .

PRESERVATION OF SEMEN AT AMBIENT AND
REFRIGERATION TEMPERATURES (Continued)

B. Name of the Dilutor

1. **Materials required**

   1. . . . .   5. . . . .
   2.   6. . . . .
   3.   7. . . . .
   4.   8. . . . .

2. **Composition of the dilutor**

3. **Extension of semen**

   Storage temperature . . . . °C

5. **Observations**

   The sperm motility in . . . . dilutor after . . . . hrs. of preservation is . . . . %

6. **Remarks**

7. **Precautions**

Signature of Student   Signature of **Instructor**

EXERCISE 12

Date . . . .

DEEP FREEZING OF SEMEN

1. **Principle**

2. **Materials required**

   1.   6. . . . .
   2.   7. . . . .
   3.   8. . . . .
   4.   9. . . . .
   5.   10. . . . .

3. **Functions of glycerol**

4. **Preparation of dilutor**

5. **Method**
   1. Semen collection and evaluation

2. Semen dilution

3. Straw filling and sealing

4. Cooling and equilibration period

5. Deep freezing

6. **Observations**
   Thawing

Motility of semen after thawing (after .... hrs. of freezing) = ... %

7. Remarks

8. Precautions

Signature of Student   **Signature of Instructor**

EXERCISE 13

Date . . . .

A.I. TECHNIQUES USING CHILLED AND FROZEN SEMEN
(RECTOVAGINAL METHOD)

1. **Check points before insemination**
    1. . . . .
    2. . . . .
    3. . . . .
    4. . . . .
    5. . . . .
    6. . . . .
2. **A.I. with liquid semen**

3. **A.I. with frozen semen (in straws)**
    1. Taking out the straw

    2. Thawing

    3. Removal of moisture from straw

4. Travel of air bubble to single plug side

5. Cutting of the straw

6. Loading of the straw in A.I. gun

7. Securing of the sheath in the A.I. gun

8. Method (rectovaginal method)
   The artificial insemination is done by rectovaginal method as described with liquid semen.
9. Site of semen deposition

4. **Remarks**

5. **Precautions**

Signature of Student   **Signature of Instructor**

EXERCISE 14

Date . . . .

PLANNING AND ORGANIZATION OF SEMEN
COLLECTION AND A.I. CENTRE

1. **Essential requirements of a bull centre**

    1. . . . .   5. . . . .

    2. . . . .   6. . . . .

    3. . . . .   7. . . . .

    4. . . . .

2. **Main considerations for the location of bull centre**

    1. . . . .

    2. . . . .

    3. . . . .

    4. . . . .

3. **Housing (bull paddock)**

		Desired	Actual
(a)	Direction	Northwest to south-east	
(b)	Area of bull house (one bull)	16′ × 16′	
(c)	Area of the open yard (one bull)	16′ × 20′	
(d)	Ceiling height	10′-12′	
(e)	Floor	Non-slippery	
(f)	Corners of bull house	Rounded	
(g)	Drainage	Sufficient slope for drainage	
(h)	Doors	Wide	

4. **Semen collection shed**

		Desired	Actual
(a)	Distance from bull house	Convenient	
(b)	Direct sunlight	No	
(c)	Dust	No	
(d)	Protection against cold and hot winds	Yes	

    (e) Protection against rain showers   Yes

    (f) Area   Sufficient

    (g) Crate   Strong, deeply burried, galvanised and provision for fastening neck

    (h) Guard rail (near crate)   Essential, suitable height and strong

—— (i) Floor   Non-slippery spread with thick layer of sand

5. Laboratory for preliminary semen examination

	Desired	Actual
(a) Location	Near to collection shed	
(b) Sliding glass window (to pass semen tube)	Yes	
(c) Lab	Clean, hygienic and dust free; good light, sufficient electric connections for equipment; good supply of water, wash basin; facility for U.V. radiation; sufficient equipment e.g. microscope, water bath, refrigerator, instrument cabinet, absorbant cotton, enameled jugs and buckets, glass wares, wash bottles, spirit lamp, aluminium foil, Eosin-Nigrosin stain, waste bucket, heater, kerosene stove, A.V. with stand etc.	

6. Store for feed and fodder

	Desired	Actual
(a) Dampness	No	
(b) Wooden planks	Yes	
(c) Protection from rats	Yes	
(d) Doors	Wide	

7. Segregation ward for sick animal

	Desired	Actual
	Clean, dry, hygienic and comfortable	

8. Facility for exercise

    Yes/No

9. **Residential quarters for attendants**   Yes/No
   If yes, whether the quarter(s) is/are at convenient distance   Yes/No
10. **A.I. shed**
    Do the animals come easily for A.I.   Yes/No
    Roof over A.I. crate   Yes/No
    A.I. crate of good quality (strong deeply burrieid, sufficient size) Yes/No
    Drainage   Good/Poor
    Distance from semen lab   Convenient/long
    Supply of water   Yes/No

11. **Remarks**

12. **Precautions**

Signature of Student   Signature of Instructor

EXERCISE 15

Date . . . .

SELECTION, CARE, TRAINING AND MAINTENANCE OF BREEDING BULLS FOR A.I.

1. **Selection criteria** (Satisfactory/Unsatisfactory) . . . .
2. **Bull's familiarity with attendants** (Yes/No) . . . .
3. **Nose ring** (Yes/No) . . . .
4. **Regular health checks** (Yes/No) . . . .
5. **Housing** (Comfortable/Not comfortable) . . . .
6. **Vaccination** (Regular/Irregular/No) . . . .
7. **De-worming** (Regular/Irregular/No) . . . .
8. **Cleaning** (Daily/Occasionally/No) . . . .
9. **Grooming/Brushing** (Daily/Occasionally/No) . . . .
10. **Clipping of prepucial hairs** (Regular/Irregular/No) . . . .
11. **Exercise to bulls** (Daily/Occasionally/No) . . . .
12. **Time of exercise** (Satisfactory/Unsatisfactory) . . . .
13. **Distance of walk** (Adequate/Less/More) . . . .
14. **Feeding** (Less/Adequate/More) . . . .
15. **Watering** (Satisfactory/Unsatisfactory) . . . .
16. **Familiarization of the bull under training to semen collection site** (Yes/No) . . . .
17. **Disturbances, if any** . . . .
18. **Semen collection time** . . . .
19. **Size of dummy** (Large/O.K./Small) . . . .
20. **Remarks**

21. **Precautions**

Signature of Student   Signature of Instructor

EXERCISE 16

Date . . . .

RECORODING SYSTEMS FOR ANDROLOGY AND A.I.

A. Semen Collection Register (Proforma)

> **Address of Semen Collection Centre**

1. Date of semen collection   . . . .
2. Yearly No.   . . . .
3. Monthly No.   . . . .
4. Bull No./Name   . . . .
5. Breed of the bull   . . . .
6. Time of semen collection   . . . .
7. Reaction time   . . . .
8. Volume of ejaculate (ml)   . . . .
9. Colour of semen   . . . .
10. Consistency of semen   . . . .
11. Mass motility   . . . .
12. Individual motility   . . . .
13. pH of the semen   . . . .
14. Live spermatozoa percentage   . . . .
15. Sperm concentration ($\times 10^6$/ml) . . . .
16. Spermatozoa abnormalities
    (a) Head abnormalities   . . . .
    (b) Middle piece abnormalities   . . . .
    (c) Tail abnormalities   . . . .
    (d) Total abnormalities   . . . .
17. Dilutor   . . . .

18. **Dilution rate** . . . .

19. **Any other significant observation** . . . .

20. **Officer's initial**

21. **Remarks**

22. **Precautions**

Signature of Student

Signature of Instructor

EXERCISE 17

Date . . . .

RECORDING SYSTEMS FOR ANDROLOGY AND A.I.

B. Bull Performance Register (Proforma)

```
+--------------------------------------------------+
|              Address of Bull Centre              |
|                                                  |
|                                                  |
|                                                  |
+--------------------------------------------------+
```

1. **Details of bull**

   Name/No. of the bull .... Date of birth/Age ....

   Breed .... Dam's yield .... Grand dam's yield ....

2. **Recording**

Date	Semen quality (Excellent/ Good/Fair)	Name of the owner	Cow/ Buffalo (No./Name)	No. of A.I. (I/II/III/ more)	Pregnancy diagnosis		Signature of Inseminator	Remarks
					Date	Result		

Overall Conception rate .... %

3. **Precautions**

Signature of Student   Signature of Instructor

EXERCISE 18

Date . . . .

RECORDING SYSTEMS FOR ANDROLOGY AND A.I.

C. Register/Individual Cards for Reproductive Records of Females (Proforma)

Address of Dairy Farm

1. **Details of female animal**
   Animal No./Name .... Date of birth/Age ....
   Breed .... Sire .... Dam ....

2. **Recording**
   1. Date of estrum   . . . .
   2. Date of A.I.   . . . .
   3. Bull No.   . . . .
   4. Semen quality (Excellent/Good/Fair/Poor)   . . . .
   5. Signature of inseminator   . . . .
   6. Date of pregnancy diagnosis with result   . . . .
   7. Calving date   . . . .
   8. Sex of calf   . . . .
   9. Weight of calf (kg)   . . . .
   10. Calving abnormality (Abortion/Dystocia/
       Retained placenta)   . . . .
   11. Other reproductive diseases (Metritis/
       Pyometra/Inactive ovaries/Cystic ovaries/
       Mummification/Maceration/Others)   . . . .
   12. Treatment   . . . .
   13. Veterinarian's Signature

3. **Remarks**

4. **Precautions**

Signature of Student   Signature of Instructor

EXERCISE 19

Date . . . .

RECORDING SYSTEMS FOR ANDROLOGY AND A.I.

D. Inseminator's Performance (Proforma)

1. **Name of the inseminator** . . . .
2. **Name of the centre** . . . .
3. **Recording**

Date of A.I.	Semen quality (Excellent/ Good/Fair/Poor)	Owner's name & address	Animal's Name/No.	Pregnancy diagnosis		Remarks
				Date	Result	

Overall performance .... %

4. **Precautions**

Signature of Student   Signature of Instructor

EXERCISE 20

Date . . . .

CARE, CLEANING, STERILIZATION, STORAGE AND UPKEEP OF EQUIPMENT USED FOR COLLECTION AND PROCESSING OF SEMEN AND A.I.

1. **Cleaning and sterilization of glass wares**

2. **Cleaning and sterilization of A.V.**

3. **Sterilization of buffer solutions**

4. **Sterilization of plastic wares**

5. **Cleaning and sterilization of laboratory**

6. **Storage of sterilized articles**
   (a) Glass wares

   (b) Catheters

   (c) Buffer solutions

   (d) A.V.

7. **Precautions**
   In cleaning

   In dry heat sterilization

   In autoclaving

   In gaseous sterilization

   In handling liquid nitrogen containers

In handling A.I. gun

In handling sheaths

In handling dip stick

Signature of Student   Signature of Instructor

Index

NOTES

NOTES

NOTES

NOTES

NOTES